ROCK
Your WORLD
NATURALLY

SEVEN DIVINE KEYS TO UNLOCK
EXTRAORDINARY HEALTH

by
Rekishia L. McMillan, MSW
Certified Integrative Nutrition Health Coach

Special Note from the Author

The information and recommendations presented within this book are based on personal experience, training, education, extensive research, and other publications pertaining to holistic health. The intent of the author is to share information that is grounded in biblical truth and scientific research to help individuals understand God's divine plan regarding holistic health and healing for the body, soul and spirit, with the most emphasis placed on physical healing. The author of this book does not prescribe the use of or discontinuance of prescription medication without the advice of a medical doctor or certified health professional. This book is not intended to replace sound medical advice from a physician. Statements within this book have not been evaluated by the Food and Drug Administration and are not intended to diagnose, prescribe, treat, or claim to prevent, mitigate, or cure any human disease. They are intended for informational and nutritional support only. The author disclaims all liability in connection with the information presented and does not recommend, endorse, or make any representation about the efficacy, appropriateness, or suitability of any specific tests, products, procedures, treatments, services, opinions, health care providers or other information that may be contained on or available within this book.

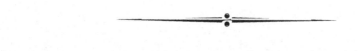

This book is dedicated to my dear mother, Stephaine Y. Nobles-Beans

You Are the Wind Beneath My Wings

Acknowledgements

To the Great Physician, Jehovah-Rapha, the Healer who has graciously given His children the keys to unlock and possess the divine promise of healing. I could never thank you enough for Your wisdom and guidance, which made it possible for me to write this book. What you have taught and shown me leaves me even more amazed at who You are. I am forever grateful and thankful. You are my world.

To my wonderful and loving parents, Johnnie Beans Sr. and Stephaine Y. Nobles-Beans. Words could never truly express how much you mean to me. Your love, prayers, strength, and resilience played a major role in shaping me into the woman that I am today. I love you. Growing up, you both had such a great influence on me regarding health and wellness. I couldn't be more elated or proud to share the gift of health with the world. I thank you deeply—for everything.

To my dear husband, Dr. Titus McMillan. You were the missing piece of the puzzle that I so desperately needed in my life. God in all of His wisdom gifted me with you. Your love has brought a sense of peace and completion that is truly heaven sent. I couldn't be more excited about our future together. The best is yet to come.

To my Aunt Wynndie. Your guidance and wisdom truly came at a time when I needed it most. I appreciate you for your prayers, love, and support to help me complete this book. You are dearly cherished and loved.

To Pastors Tolbert and Lady Philicia Blacknall. I graciously thank you for all that you have imparted into my life personally and spiritually. You and the Bethel family will always have a special place in my heart.

To my son Kishon. You are my Superstar! Thank you for always being there to listen to my many health stories. Even when I've worn your ear out with them, you still listen. Thank you for encouraging me to keep pressing forward to write this book. Mom loves you beyond words.

To my dearly beloved siblings: Leola, Cliff, Johnnie Jr., Natasha, Stephaine, and Jason. I could not have prayed for more loving siblings than you. Not only are you my sisters and brothers, you are my best friends. I love you.

To all of the natural healers who have come before me, upon whose shoulders I stand. If there was ever a time to return to the ways of God to heal our world, it is now. Thank you.

Table of Contents

Preface...**15**
   The Current System 15
   Where Does the Healthcare System Stand?....................16
   What is Rock Your World Naturally? 17
   It's Time to Use Your Keys 17
   We Are in a Battle to Stay Healthy 18
   It's Time to Slay the Giants.....................................18
   We Have the Weapons to Win 19
   Be Open-minded 21
   Be Patient with Yourself...22
   Practice, Practice and More Practice............................22

Chapter 1 – In the Beginning..**23**
   My Journey 23
   Christian Psychology 26
   Blood and Your Health..27
   The Cycle 28
   How Do Toxins Contaminate Your Bloodstream?...........29
   In the Beginning...30
   Paradise Lost...30
   The Industrial Revolution 31

Chapter 2 – Fresh Air and Your Health..................................**35**
   Why Fresh Air is Crucial 36
   Why Getting Outside in Green Spaces Matters 37
   You Must Know About Jennie Camuto 38
   Add More Green Space to Your World 39
   Vitamin D and Green Spaces 39

Fresh Air: A Cure for Cancer?...40

The Dangers of Being Surrounded by Enclosed Spaces..........40

Are Indoor Spaces Making You Sick? 41

Sick Building Syndrome (SBS) 42

Toxins Are in Found in Every Day Products 44

Technology and Unhealthy Lifestyle Habits 46

You Must Get Up and Out, It's Time to Move…Exercise,

    Exercise, Exercise 47

Inhalation and Mercury Fillings..48

Alternative Solution to Mercury Fillings 49

Breathing and Deepening Your Consciousness 50

Let's Get Back to the Beginning 51

Chapter 3 - Learn to Love the Skin That You're In **57**

Just How Important is Your Skin? 58

So…What's the Problem with Personal Care Products?..........59

What's Actually In My Personal Care Products?.....................60

Wake Up Before It's Too Late..61

Skin Absorption and the Internal War 61

Autoimmune Disorders Are On the Rise 62

A Special Word on Beauty 63

It's Time to Begin Thinking Critically 65

Why Are Chemical Laced Products Allowed to Be Sold? . . .65

Use Products that Are Safe For Your Skin 66

Change the Law by Letting Your Voice Be Heard 67

Being a Good Steward of Your Temple....................................69

Chapter 4 - What You Are Injecting into Your World? **73**

Tattoos and You...74

Tattoos and Spiritual implications...75

Tattoos and Health Implications..76

The Real Fountain of Youth... 77

Botox is Highly Toxic.. 81

Are Vaccinations Dangerous? 82

Build Up Your Immune System 86

Making Wise Choices to Protect Your Skin 89

**Chapter 5 - Is What You're Eating Wrecking
Your Healthy World?** **93**
What is Food? 93
The Industrial Revolution Changed Our Relationship
with Food 94
Garbage In, Garbage Out 94
Processed Foods and Your Health.................................... 95
Pesticides & Your Food...96
Alternatives to Pesticide Produce.....................................97
How to Shop for Organic Produce 97
What Are Genetically Modified Organism (GMO) Foods? . . 99
Why Are Companies Producing GMO's?.......................... 100
GMO's and Our World 101
GMO's and Our Environment..101
GMO's and Your Health...102
Why Eating Humanely Raised Meat Matters.......................106
Genetically Engineered Meat and Fish 108
It's Time to Change the Law..108
Eating Is a Spiritual Practice 109
It's Time to Think About What You Are Eating....................110
How We Are Eating Is Important......................................112
Eating and Your Blood Type Diet 113
God's Way is Always the Best Way.................................. 114

Chapter 6 - Water: The Essential Nutrient for Life....................**119**
Water is a Vital Nutrient..120
Americans Are Simply Not Drinking Enough Water 122
Choosing Flavor Over Health 123
The Problem with Consuming Too Much Sugar................... 124
It's Time to Upgrade Your Fuel..124
The Effects of Sugar on Your Blood Cells...........................125
Do Not Despise the Blessing of Water 126
How Much Water Do You Need to Drink? 127
Hot, Cold, or Room Temperature...What Is the Best Way to
Drink Water? 129
God Always Has a Purpose 130
Why I'm Not a Fan of Bottled Water 131

How Safe Is Bottled Water?.. 131
How Much Is Bottled Water Costing Our Nation? 132
Alternative to Drinking Bottled Water 134
Bring Your Own Bottled Water 135
There's Healing in the Water.................................. 135

Chapter 7 - Why Essential Oils Are a Must in Your World 139
Our First Medicine..139
What Are Essential Oils? 140
Essential Oils and the Bible 141
The Importance of Using Quality Essential Oils 148
How Do They Work?.. 149
Essential Oils and Your Bloodstream......................150
Dollars Over Health 151
The Straight Facts About Prescription Medications.............152
The More Excellent Way 153
Hospitals Are Beginning to Follow God's Original
    Blueprint 153
Breaking Away from the American Way 153
We Must Change Our Approach 154

Chapter 8 – Remember the Sabbath 161
The Sabbath 162
History of the Sabbath 162
Christians and the Sabbath.....................................164
Our Nation is Spinning Out of Control....................165
We Need a Remedy...166
My Experience 167
How Did America Become So Busy?........................168
It's Time to Make An Adjustment............................169
The Concepts of Rhythm and Time.........................170
What Happens to the Body During Sleep? 170
America is a Sleep Deprived and Overworked Nation 171
How Much Sleep Do You Really Need?....................172
The Intent of Remembering the Sabbath 173

Chapter 9 - Protecting and Preserving Planet Earth................**179**

    The Earth is Alive 182

    Stewardship Over the Earth 183

    Printed vs. Electronic Receipts 184

    Reusable Bags vs. Paper and Plastic Bags 185

    Ditching the Plastic Bag.. 186

    Food Miles and Our Health..187

    The Benefits of Growing Your Own Food 188

    Why it Pays to Buy Your Food Locally 189

    Mindless Consumption 189

    Choose Whole Food Over Packaged, Boxed, Canned, or

        Bottled Food...191

    Paper Towels & Paper Napkins Are Way Overrated!............191

    How Much Are Paper Products Costing Us? 192

    A Call to Responsible Stewardship 193

Chapter 10 - Will You Join the Health Revolution? **199**

Rock Your World

*[The ability to make an extraordinary
eternal impact into the personal world of
another encompassing body, soul, and spirit]*

Naturally

*[Having, constituting, or relating to a
classification based on features
stemming from God's original
creation or nature]*

*Rock Your World Naturally is a natural way of achieving
extraordinary health from the inside out. It is a lifestyle
designed to raise your consciousness to a higher
level of living physically, spiritually, emotionally, and
environmentally.*

Rock Your World Naturally

Behold, I will bring it health and cure, and I will cure them, and will reveal unto them the abundance of peace and truth.
Jeremiah 33:6

Preface

The Current System

You don't need to go very far to realize that individuals are facing health challenges all around us. Depression, auto-immune disorders, excessive weight, stress, low energy, no sex drive, irregular blood sugar, chronic fatigue, hormonal imbalance, aches, and pains are continually at the forefront of daily living. If it's not you, it's a family member, friend, co-worker or neighbor. Trillions of dollars are funneled annually into the healthcare system to improve physical well-being, yet, increased spending is not equating to better health. On the contrary, chronic illness is multiplying at an all-time high and has become the new normal in American culture.

Healthcare spending in the United States is more than 2.6 trillion each year, and more than half of that money spent is wastefully [1]. A study published by the Dartmouth Institute for Health Policy and Clinical Practice reveals that up to one-third of wasteful spending is attributed to unnecessary hospitalizations, redundant tests, unproven treatments, and excessive end-of-life care [2,3]. These inefficient methods often leave individuals with even more health complications than they had prior to seeing their doctors.

Where Does the Healthcare System Stand?

The United States boasts of having the best medical treatment and healthcare system in the world, however, countless reports note that America ranks number one in having the most chronically ill individuals out of all countries. In fact, the United States ranks last among eleven developed countries in delivery, coordination, and equality of healthcare [4]. Millions of Americans are diagnosed annually with heart disease, cancer, obesity, mental health disorders, and diabetes. The list of new diseases keeps growing, as do the statistics associated with poor health. This begs the question of the efficacy of the healthcare system: is what we have in place really working?

> *Is there no balm in Gilead? Is there no physician there?*
> *Why then has not the health of the daughter of my people*
> *been restored?*
>
> *Jeremiah 8:22*

Personally, I have been treated and helped by some of the most wonderful physicians. I am thankful to God for those serving in the medical profession, because they are making a difference. In no way do I fault healthcare professionals or practitioners for the ineffectiveness of the system, but what I do question are the conventional methods that are utilized to treat and address individual health needs. The current model is guided by a one-size-fits-all business approach, focusing primarily on the short-term treatment of symptoms rather than investigating the root cause of illness to bring about long-term healing for life. This business model approach has resulted in more and more patients leaving their doctors' offices with no definitive answers. When enormous out-of-pocket expenses, disproportionate co-pays, and bureaucratic red tape involving medical insurance coverage are factored in, it's enough to leave any person feeling frustrated, confused, hopeless, and discouraged. If you or a loved one is diagnosed with a life-threatening disease, this is not the kind of health "care" that anyone deserves. We are living in an unprecedented time where people no longer want to operate within this type of system. They are desperately seeking different solutions to experience better health and an improved quality of life, and Rock Your World Naturally provides such an alternative.

What is Rock Your World Naturally?

Rock Your World Naturally is natural way of achieving extraordinary health from the inside out. It is a lifestyle designed to raise your consciousness to a higher level of living physically, spiritually, emotionally, and environmentally. To be clear, Rock Your World Naturally is not based on the latest diet fad or passing trend, but firmly rests upon seven key principles that are founded upon the truth of God's infallible Word. When fully embraced, these seven keys will bring balance into every area of your personal world. These divine keys will empower you to use preventative and maintenance based approaches according to your unique health needs.

> *Jesus said, "And I will give unto thee the keys of the Kingdom of Heaven: and whatsoever thou shalt bind on earth shall be bound in Heaven: and whatsoever thou shalt loose on earth shall be loosed in Heaven."*
>
> *Matthew 18:19*

It's Time to Use Your Keys

As Jesus spoke these words to Peter, the keys that He spoke of represented three of the greatest gifts that God has given to His sons and daughters. First, our Lord and Savior Jesus Christ has given us authority. Second, we have been endowed with the power of the Holy Spirit to lead and assist us on the earth, and third, we have been given dominion over the earth and everything in it, including our health.

> *Trust in the Lord with all your heart and lean not on your own understanding; in all your ways submit to him, and he will make your paths straight. Do not be wise in your own eyes; fear the Lord and shun evil.*
>
> *Proverbs 3:5-7*

For too long, we have trusted in faulty systems and methods rather than relying on God's principles regarding our health. As a result, our health has been locked up, because we have not used our keys to access the promises associated with divine health. In God's Kingdom, there is no sickness. His will has always been that we live and walk according to 3 John 2, "Beloved, I pray that you may prosper in every way and [that your body] may keep well, even as [I know] your soul keeps well and prospers. Now is the time for Christians to return to God's original plan concerning health. By understanding and applying the seven keys, you will be equipped with tools that will serve as the first line of defense to help you begin taking ownership of your health. Over time you will learn how to listen to and understand what your body needs to stay strong, balanced, and healthy.

I've been blessed to assist family members, friends, and clients on their journey to creating a healthier personal world by incorporating these keys into their everyday life. I've come to understand that most individuals simply don't know where to begin or what to do to improve their health. Simply put, they lack knowledge. Like many others, once you apply the knowledge associated with the seven keys, over time, you can begin feeling more confident, strong, liberated, focused, happy, and healthy. You can transition into the way that God desires for you to move in the world.

We Are in a Battle to Stay Healthy

People from all walks of life are entangled in fierce and intense warfare, spiritually, and physically, fighting to maintain or regain the divine health that God has promised. Every day we are faced with invisible and intangible giants that challenge our health on every hand. The giants overshadowing America are a broken health care system, an overabundance of unhealthy foods, the excessive use of prescription medication, the never-ending roller coaster of diet trends, unhealthy lifestyle habits, and corporations driven by financial greed flooding our grocery stores, schools, and homes with toxic food and products. These giants have a synergistic strategy designed to keep Gods' people trapped in an unhealthy and debilitating state. Is it possible to stand up against these giants? The answer is yes!

It's Time to Slay the Giants

Are you familiar with the story of David and Goliath? In I Samuel 17, Goliath is described as a 9-foot tall Philistine giant that tormented David's country day and night. He was known as a battle-hardened soldier that vanquished anyone who dared to cross his path. Goliath was quite intimidating, giving David's country no rest as he spewed out negative words and harsh threats about enslaving their nation. Goliath challenged someone to fight him, and whichever side won, their country would become enslaved to the other. No one was brave enough to accept his challenge or stand up to the giant, not the king or any of the other valiant warriors. The bible says the men of Israel became afraid and ran off.

While the standoff between Goliath and Israel took place, David was sent on an errand by his father to carry lunch to his brothers who were on the battlefield. As David came upon the encampment, he couldn't avoid overhearing the loud threats that were being made by the sinister giant. What David saw and heard filled his heart with deep concern. As he talked with some of the men, he discovered that king Saul had placed an offer on the table: the man who slays the giant will be given great riches, the king's daughter to marry, and his father's house would be free from paying taxes. What a reward! After hearing this, David asks the men, "Who is this uncircumcised Philistine that he should defy the armies of the living God?" David's oldest brother overheard him and became angry with him for inquiring about the giant and told him to go back into the fields to tend his sheep in the wilderness. In return, David replied, "Is there not a cause?"

David was a young shepherd boy whose only battle experience had taken place while tending sheep on two separate occasions. When his precious sheep were threatened with attacks from a lion and a bear, David single-handedly killed both animals. Surely, if he had killed a lion and a bear, he could conquer Goliath. With great faith, David accepted his challenge and withstood Goliath with no fancy armor or weaponry. He was confident in the God who had been with him in the past and believed that He would not fail him now. David's weapons were five smooth stones, plain, and simple, yet with only one stone, David killed Goliath, bringing freedom and justice to the land.

We Have the Weapons to Win

Analogous to the story of David and Goliath, the giant systems that are confronting our health are becoming increasingly louder, more boisterous and ever-present, as they vie to keep men, women, and children enslaved in a world of sickness and disease. Just as David presented his brothers and the men of Israel with the question, "is there not a cause?" You too have a cause, a reason to fight for your health. God's will for His church is to live an abundant life that includes being and feeling healthy. As a child of God, you must possess the necessary zeal, energy, drive, and creative ability to fully carry out the tasks and assignments that God has specifically designed for you to complete on earth. This is the reason why you must stand up to slay the giants that are fighting against your health. If we are not feeling well physically, we will not be able to effectively accomplish much of anything. Just as David used something as simple and basic as a smooth stone to slay the giant, the same posture can be applied to the seven keys associated with the Rock Your World Naturally lifestyle. The keys are simplistic in nature, yet powerful enough to provide you with a God-centered strategy to radically improve your health and quality of life. As you read this book, you'll discover:

- Seven biblical keys to unlock extraordinary divine health

- The relationship between your blood cells and health

- What external forces are wrecking your healthy world

- What is causing you to spin off of your personal axis

- How to bring your world back into balance naturally

- How to embrace the Rock Your World Naturally lifestyle for a lifetime

We can no longer entrust our health to unreliable systems that have proven to be ineffective and complicated. Our bodies have been deemed as temples of the Living God, and as such, He has entrusted each of us to be good and faithful stewards over our bodies. You have been charged with the personal responsibility to protect, maintain, and preserve the precious gift of health that rightfully belongs to you.

My mission is to serve as your health and wellness ambassador by educating, motivating, challenging, and encouraging you to transform your current world into the world that God has destined for you; a world that is overflowing with vibrant health, happiness, love, peace, and abundance. Overcoming health challenges is possible when you possess the right tools and information. It is important to understand that experiencing abundant health does not just happen for "faith without works is dead" (James 2:26). Restoring your health is a journey that requires prayer, patience, diligence, and effort on your part. Unfortunately, some people are not willing to work for their success. However, if you are willing to pay the price, God's promise of living in extraordinary health belongs to you.

> *Health transformation begins with having an open mind, patience, and practice. The effort you put forth is a small price to pay for the long-term rewards. Regaining your divine health is priceless.*

As you read this book, I ask that you to do three things:

1) Have an open mind
2) Be patient
3) Practice what you are learning

Be Open-minded

You may be someone who has relied on old methods stemming from the health care system that are not working. Because this is the only way that you have been accustomed to practicing for most of your life, it can seem a little daunting or even strange to try something new. I'll admit, when I first began my journey towards achieving better health, what I learned was very different than what I was familiar with. As I embraced this new way, I became very open to alternative practices and when I did, I began to see major changes regarding my health. In actuality, the ways that I learned were not new, but were always what God had planned from the beginning of time. By reading this book, it lets me know that you are eager and ready for change. So, remember to keep an open mind.

Be Patient with Yourself

It took years for your health to deteriorate and it will take time and patience to fully restore your health. Solomon's temple was not built overnight. It took time and likewise, it will take time for you to rebuild your temple. Life is journey and a true gift from God. One that must be travelled one day at a time, one step at a time, one prayer at a time. Oftentimes, your personal health journey may seem challenging and require you to take the road less travelled. You can rest assured in knowing that the roads ordained by God will lead you into places of richness that are filled with greener pastures and still peaceful waters. Rely on God's strength as you make the effort to change and move forward.

> *I have strength for all things in Christ Who empowers me [I am ready for anything and equal to anything through Him Who infuses inner strength into me; I am self-sufficient in Christ's sufficiency].*
>
> *Philippians 4:13*

Practice, Practice and More Practice

Please do not let this be just another book that you read and take no action on. The information in this book will be of no benefit to you if you do not apply it. Consistently practicing healthy habits over time leads to a healthy lifestyle.

> *Your beliefs become your thoughts,*
> *Your thoughts become your words,*
> *Your words become your actions,*
> *Your actions become your habits,*
> *Your habits become your values,*
> *Your values become your destiny.*
>
> *Mahatma Gandhi*

Now that you have an idea of what's in store, are you ready for the adventure? Ready... Set... Go! It's time to ***Rock Your World Naturally!***

To Your Health and Happiness,
Rekishia

"The life of any creature is in the blood."
Leviticus 17:11

Chapter 1

In the Beginning

·❖·

My Journey

If you are like most people, your story may be similar to mine. A few years back, I suffered from a number of health conditions that included Chronic Fatigue Syndrome, Major Depressive Disorder, Myalgia (a form of Fibromyalgia), Degenerative Disks, Fibroids, Candida Overgrowth Syndrome, Hypoglycemia, and a near bout with Lyme's disease after being bitten by a tick. By personally experiencing each of these conditions, I learned a great deal about how God created the human body. It has the amazing ability to heal itself when provided with the right nutrients and self-care aids.

I gained greater insight and came to understand that just because we are Christians, does not mean we are exempt from facing health challenges. While it is true that we are created in the image and likeness of our Father as tri-part beings, possessing a spirit, soul, and body, we live and operate in the physical realm. Walking in divine health requires that we abide within the laws of health to stay physically well. Naturally, if you violate a traffic law, there is a consequence. Depending on what kind of violation it is, the fine or penalty can be quite hefty. So it is with our health, if we violate the laws of health, negative repercussions are inevitable.

From the beginning of creation, God has always had a specific plan of health for us to follow. Throughout the bible, He gave detailed laws about eating, rest, cleansing, prayer, and fasting. In Hosea 4:6 we are reminded, "My people are destroyed for lack of knowledge: because you have rejected knowledge, I will also reject you, that you shall be no priest to me: because you have forgotten the law of your God, I will also forget your children." The words spoken through the prophet Hosea are very firm and harsh because God wanted the children of Israel to understand that when you move away from God's original plan or design, the results are never fruitful and impact not only you, but future generations.

I'm convinced that one of the main reasons why we are experiencing so much sickness in the world today is because we have moved far away from and discarded God's original plan for our health. Unfortunately, these choices are also adversely affecting our children. The Father created natural and spiritual laws in order to provide healthy boundaries that ensure our protection and well-being, certainly not to deny us of anything. God knows the plans that He has for you, plans to help you prosper and not to harm you, plans to give you hope and a future (Jeremiah 29:11).

Like so many others, I was taught to rely solely on the conventional wisdom to help me get well when faced with health challenges. After visiting doctor after doctor and being prescribed one prescription after another, there was no permanent change in any of my health conditions. In fact, I felt worse depending on which medication I took and which physician I visited last.

Many weekends, I remember being so fatigued that I could barely eat, and all I wanted to do was sleep. Instead of improving and feeling better, I grew worse and experienced a downward spiral. This gravely impacted my personal life and my ability to care for my son, who was 5 years old at the time. My health was affected in such a way that my mother had my youngest sister move in with me to help me take care of my son. Every day was a challenge and I could barely make it through each day. Most days, I felt like a walking zombie. There were days that it would take me three hours or more to get out and bed because my energy levels were extremely low.

When I did muster up enough strength to get up, I would sit on the edge of my bed in tears because I felt so horrible. Every morning I would wake up feeling like I had been hit by a ton of bricks and was heavily weighed down. *"This is no way for a woman in her early thirties to feel,"* I would think to myself, *"I'm too young for this."* Because I was not feeling well physically, it impacted my life spiritually, and I was not as effective as I could have been in my service to the Kingdom of God. It was a struggle for me to have regular fellowship time with God in prayer, studying, or reading my bible; it was like climbing Mount Kilimanjaro. Although I was applying my faith through prayer, physically I did not feel any different. Still, I believed that God would change my physical well-being. On one occasion, after visiting my doctor she told me, "Rekishia your blood work looks like that of an athlete." I looked at her and said, "Doctor if that's the case, why do I feel so bad? Why do I feel like I've been hit by a sledgehammer when I wake up every morning?"

As usual, we went over the symptoms that I was exhibiting. I was chronically fatigued, extremely depressed, and could not focus on tasks for extended periods of time. I was highly sensitive to harsh chemicals and perfumes, which felt very disorienting. I asked, "Doctor what is going on with me physically?" She gently smiled and said, "Look at your blood work, the test results are all normal. They are some of the best that I've seen. Don't worry, you'll be fine." With no substantial answers for me, she filled out another prescription, medicating the symptoms for something that could not be identified instead of treating the root cause.

On a different occasion, another one of my doctors said, "There's nothing wrong with you, it's all in your head. Maybe you need to speak to someone." Because of my background in clinic therapy work, I knew that what I was experiencing was not a condition that needed to be treated with psychotherapy alone. This was something physical, not mental, but I did not know what to do or how to go about it. I often wondered why my doctors, who were board certified and trained in medicine, didn't know how to help me. When I felt like I was at my lowest point physically, mentally, spiritually, and emotionally, I remember praying for a major change. Finally, I received the answers from God that I had been desperately longing for. What I discovered were simple and natural ways of reversing the illnesses that were plaguing my world. It totally Rocked My World Naturally!

God revealed in Leviticus 17:11, that the health, strength, energy, and vitality of all living creatures, begins and ends with our blood cells. In order for me to feel better, my blood cells needed a healthy environment to thrive in. There were several factors impeding my health that stemmed from the environment, my eating choices and lifestyle habits. Unbeknownst to me, these factors were making my bloodstream toxic and wreaking havoc on my immune system, thus creating improper imbalances within my body. The toxins in my bloodstream were the root cause of my health issues. I needed a plan of action to remove these toxins from my body, a process also known as detoxification or detox. God created our bodies to naturally rid itself of toxins, but when your body reaches a point of toxic overload, the process is hindered and places an extreme burden on your body. As God revealed the underlying cause of my health problems, I began using the seven keys, which you will learn about in this book. Through faith and patience, my body became balanced, my strength and energy levels returned and I began feeling good again—amazing, actually.

Christian Psychology

As I physically recovered from the different illness that were impacting my health, the Holy Spirit reminded me about what the Apostle Paul wrote to the Body of Christ in Romans 12:1-2 (Amp).

> *I appeal to you therefore, brethren, and beg of you in view of [all] the mercies of God, to make a decisive dedication of your bodies [presenting all your members and faculties] as a living sacrifice, holy (devoted, consecrated) and well pleasing to God, which is your reasonable (rational, intelligent) service and spiritual worship. Do not be conformed to this world (this age), [fashioned after and adapted to its external, superficial customs], but be transformed (changed) by the [entire] renewal of your mind [by its new ideals and its new attitude], so that you may prove [for yourselves] what*

*is the good and acceptable and perfect will of God, even
the thing which is good and acceptable and perfect [in
His sight for you].*

God has a method that is radically different from the world's system to care for our physical bodies. Often, when we hear about or read this passage of scripture it is equated to our dedication to Christian service, attending church regularly, showing the love of Christ or being involved in the community, but rarely is this passage taken into consideration regarding the laws and principles surrounding health.

By experiencing my health challenges, I learned that the overwhelming majority of physicians who practice traditional medicine are not trained or educated about environmental and food toxins and their effects on the bloodstream. If medical personnel are educated in these areas, the health care system does provide the necessary tools to address it. It was through prayer, faith, patience and education that God revealed what   I was experiencing. This taught me a valuable lesson, that although medical personnel are in place, they do not hold all of the answers. They are in fact "practicing" medicine based upon the system that they have been educated by.

I had to renew my psychology towards new ideals and God-centered attitudes that were drastically different than the way that I had been trained and taught to think about health all of my life. I had to learn how to trust in the Lord with all of my heart and lean not to my own understanding, acknowledging Him in all of my ways, allowing Him to direct my pathway (Proverbs 3:5). Because the health of our blood is the requisite for excellent health, the predominant theme of this book will rest on this premise. Having a healthy bloodstream is the crux upon which all the seven keys to experiencing extraordinary health hinge.

Blood and Your Health

The blood, also known as the "River of Life," is comprised of red blood cells, which carry oxygen; white blood cells that fight off infection and disease; and plasma, the liquid solution that carries everything [1]. These components work harmoniously with our vital organs to achieve optimal levels of health. The chief responsibility of the blood is to serve as the body's transport system, carrying oxygen and essential nutrients to our brain, lungs, heart, liver, pancreas, and kidneys [2]. The blood also carries waste products and eliminates carbon dioxide through the lungs. Every day, the body needs a new supply of fresh red blood cells to replace old cells that have been broken down.

> *Having a clean bloodstream that is free from toxins is one of the most significant elements to maintaining your health. Clean oil is to the car is as clean blood to the body.*

Anyone who has been driving for a while knows that your car will not last very long if you do not change the oil at a reasonable frequency. Depending on your vehicle, oil is usually changed every 3,000 to 5,000 miles. Adding clean oil to your car does not remove contaminates in the existing oil. In order for your car to run smoothly, a clean, fresh supply of oil must replace the dirty oil.

If your oil is not changed, some of the problems that can arise from having dirty oil are: engine breakdown, reduced engine life, decrease in gasoline mileage, and rough engine performance. Conversely, clean oil reduces engine friction, removes engine sludge, lowers the engines operating temperatures and ensures the proper maintenance and longevity of your car. Similar to vehicle maintenance, when red blood cells are not replenished and toxins are not released, consequently, your body slowly begins to break down, exhibiting rough and poor performance. Various symptoms in the form of sluggishness, headaches, irritability, aches, pains, and other illnesses begin to manifest. Because clean blood to the body is as clean oil to a car, it is imperative to develop a regular maintenance system to keep your bloodstream free of toxins. If a clean bloodstream is such an essential component to our health, why isn't it integrated as a primary factor within the health care model?

The Cycle

Prior to becoming a health educator, I did not truly realize or understand the importance of health maintenance regarding the blood. When I was facing health challenges, doctors did complete my blood work, however, it didn't go much farther than reading my blood cell counts or LDL levels, both of which are important, but that was about it. I felt like I was caught up in a mechanical routine that never seemed to change that looked something like this:

1. Not Feeling Well
2. Visit My Doctor
3. Receive a Prescription
4. Leave Feeling the Same or Worse
5. Repeat the Same Cycle Over Again

I went through this cycle for about seven years, and knew that deep down there had to be another way. Like me, most people are caught up in this same cycle. They are following the current health care model, but there is no permanent change in their health. This is because the root of our health, and the various factors associated with toxins in the blood are not considered.

Just like the oil in your car becomes contaminated, your bloodstream also becomes contaminated because it exposed to thousands of external toxins every day. The presence of toxins in the body damages blood cells, compromises the immune system, and eventually produces sickness and disease [3]. Psalms 103 outlines many of the benefits that we are entitled to, with one of them being physical health. God has given of this wonderful promise, and in order to tightly secure it, we must be aware of the multitude of toxins that can rob and destroy our health.

How Do Toxins Contaminate Your Bloodstream?

Scientific research has proven that toxins found in the bloodstream enter the body in 4 different ways:

1) What we breath in - **Inhalation**
2) Substances that penetrate the skin - **Absorption**
3) What we eat and drink - **Ingestion**
4) When our skin is pierced by an object - **Injection**

You might be wondering; how can these common routines impact my health in such a negative way? In the beginning, it was not this way.

Toxins are prevalent today are a result of circumstances that initially took place in the Garden of Eden.

In the Beginning

When God created the heavens and the earth, the world that He gave to us was toxin free. The earth was overflowing with pristine rivers, clean streams, and pure oceans—perfect environments for plant and sea life to thrive. God gave Adam dominion over the fowl of the air, and over the cattle and over all the earth and over every living thing that moved and crawled upon the face of the earth (Gen. 1:26). After completing His creation, God saw everything that He had made and said that it was very good (Gen. 1:31). It was the perfect paradise where God walked and talked with Adam in the cool of the day (Gen. 3:8).

I imagine that during one of their evening walks, God had a conversation with Adam to teach him how to interact with the earth. He probably explained how the earth would provide an abundant supply of food, fresh water, and adequate shelter for him and his family. He taught Adam that because he had been given dominion over the earth, it was a gift from God to be respected and cared for. Use only the resources that you need, leave the land as you found it, and take care of the things that the earth provided. This was a special time in history that was not only beautiful, but short-lived.

Paradise Lost

After the fall of man in the Garden of Eden, sin entered into the earth and Adam would now be required to work by the sweat of his brow (Gen. 3:19). No longer would he take walks with the Father in the cool of the day to receive wisdom, guidance, and instructions on how to live in oneness with the earth. Now, Adam had to rely on his own wisdom, the wisdom of man.

This world's wisdom is foolishness in God's sight
I Corinthians 3:19b

Whenever we step outside the bounds that God has established for our lives, the price that we must pay often comes at a great cost. The sins of Adam and Eve made the earth vulnerable to becoming spiritually and environmentally toxic. In Genesis 3:17, the bible says that because of sin, the land or ground became cursed and began growing thorns and thistles, representing a chaotic and unstable state. This same pattern of environmental unrest and toxicity is prevalent on the earth today, but only in a greater measure, most notably with the inception of the Industrial Revolution.

The Industrial Revolution

The massive influx of environmental toxins erupted with the Industrial Revolution, which began in the mid-1700s in England and around the mid-1800s in the United States [4]. This monumental shift in societal structure catapulted America from being an agrarian culture to one of industrial domination. The widespread use of machines replaced hundreds of jobs that were once completed by human labor. With the promise of new jobs and higher wages, agricultural families uprooted their loved ones from rural farmlands to become a part of this new way of life. In Tower of Babel like fashion, and as if overnight, skyscrapers, machinery, factories, refineries, cars, trains, and trucks sprawled up across the United States, quickly populating the country's landscape. All of which contributed to environmental toxins.

> *Then they said, "Come, let us build ourselves a city, with a tower that reaches to the heavens, so that we may make a name for ourselves; otherwise we will be scattered over the face of the whole earth." But the Lord came down to see the city and the tower the people were building. The Lord said, "If as one people speaking the same language they have begun to do this, then nothing they plan to do will be impossible for them."*
>
> *Genesis 11:4-6*

Industrialized communities were able to generate and transport food, medicine, and clothing on much larger scales by air, land, and sea quickly and efficiently. Although this transformation is considered a major milestone in our history, the grave outcomes associated with human health and the preservation of our environment were not fully comprehended. Century's later, industrial practices have not changed and have dramatically increased in supply, demand, transport, and in the production of goods.

While the Industrial Revolution advanced technological development, the consequent toxic threats affecting human health and environmental safety cannot be ignored.

In the following chapters, the impact of toxins and the health of the blood will be explored beginning with the first of the seven keys relating to fresh air and the life of our blood cells.

Key # 1

Supply Your Body with Fresh Air
Through Exercise and
Healthy Lifestyle Habits

[Inhalation / the process of
breathing in air]

Let everything that has breath
praise the Lord!

Psalms 150:6

The doctor of the future will give no medicine, but will involve the patient in the proper use of food, fresh air and exercise.
Thomas Edison

Chapter 2

Fresh Air and Your Health

O ut of all of the elements earth, water, fire, and air – air is the cornerstone of human existence. Adam took his very first breath of fresh air when God breathed the breath of life into his nostrils, causing him to become a living soul (Gen. 2:7). We can survive for weeks without food and even a few days without water, but only a few minutes without air. In this chapter, I'll explain the natural function of breathing and the significance associated with why you must get an adequate supply of fresh air to keep your body healthy. I'll also provide some beneficial breathing tools to aid you in developing rituals to improve and enhance your health. Besides, what could be more natural than breathing?

Breathing is a process that we don't give much thought to. God divinely created our bodies to perform this automatic function day in and day out. When we inhale fresh air, oxygen enters the lungs and moves throughout the blood. Breathing is responsible for several vital functions, which include: supplying our kidneys and brain with oxygen-rich blood, removing toxins like carbon dioxide from the body, regulating physiological and psychological functions, balancing our nervous and circulatory systems, and controlling our metabolism [1]. On the other hand, if the body does not receive adequate amounts of oxygen from fresh air our health begins to deteriorate.

> *Since oxygen was one of the first elements created by God to regulate and sustain the human body, it must be one of the primary areas of focus when addressing illness and physical health.*

Why Fresh Air is Crucial

Empirical studies have proven that not supplying the body with adequate amounts of fresh air can result in oxygen deficiency and is linked to many health problems [2, 3.]

- Brain injury

- Depression

- Chronic fatigue

- Dullness of mind

- Drowsiness

- Irritability

- Seizures

- Elevated blood pressure

- Confusion

- Headaches

- Insomnia

- Restlessness

- Psychological problems

- Neurological problems

- Cellular damage which can lead to cancer and other chronic illnesses

To determine if you are oxygen deficient, you can consult your doctor to have him or her measure your current oxygen levels. Consistently nourishing our bodies with fresh air is not a topic of discussion that receives much attention, however this key is crucial to our overall health.

Healthcare providers are automatically trained to prescribe medications to treat symptoms that could very well be associated with oxygen deficiency. Imagine if we took a different approach to health care. Instead of automatically prescribing medications for migraines, insomnia, attention disorders, low energy or depression, what if physicians substituted it with a natural lifestyle prescription: get out into the fresh air at least 5 times a week for a minimum of 30 minutes. This is one of the most basic, yet highly effective keys to health and healing at the cellular level.

> *But God has chosen the small, simple things to confound the wisdom of man.*
>
> *Corinthians 1:27*

You might be asking, could something as simple as creating a routine practice of being outside and getting fresh air really improve my health? Yes, and here's why.

Why Getting Outside in Green Spaces Matters

One of the things that I love most about living in New Jersey is that is filled with an abundance of green space i.e. wooded areas, biking trails, parks, and hiking trails. I make a point of spending quality time outside as much as possible because I understand the importance of flooding my body with fresh air. Have you ever noticed how your body feels when get out into the fresh air after feeling sluggish or tired? Naturally, you feel more energized and refreshed because your body is getting a much-needed supply of oxygen.

Individuals who spend adequate amounts of time in green space experience less anxiety and depression than those who live in industrial areas. On average, studies show that the concentration of salivary cortisol, a stress hormone, in people who walk through or look upon forest scenery or green spaces for 20 minutes is 13.4 percent lower than that of people in urban settings [4]. Do you remember learning about the process of photosynthesis in grade school? If not, here's a refresher. Basically, when sunlight touches green leaves, the leaves convert the light into energy and the leaves release oxygen into the atmosphere. Photosynthesis not only supplies most of the energy necessary for life on earth, this process also provides us with an oxygen-rich environment to nourish our blood cells.

You Must Know About Jennie Camuto

I am convinced that one of the reasons why my 93-year old neighbor, Jennie Camuto, is still enjoying a long and healthy life is because she takes time to sit outside and enjoy the fresh air and sunshine. Jennie still cooks, takes care of herself, eats healthy, cleans her own home, is sharp mentally and loves to read. On many days, when I pull up into my driveway, I find her sitting outside on her porch reading a good book. I can't help but join her. Jennie has had an amazing effect on my community in her very own way. When she starts out, Jennie is usually sitting alone outside, but just before the sun sets, one or more neighbors gathers on her porch. They sit in their chairs, talking, laughing, sharing stories, and enjoying the fresh air. About three years ago, you would see Jennie and her husband Frank, sitting outside together. He was 94 years old and they were married for more than 70 years before he passed away after a fall. I share their story because they are living examples of how getting out in the fresh air consistently can aid in leading a long and healthy life.

Add More Green Space to Your World

The healing and restorative effects of being in green space are indispensable to preserving your health. The many benefits stemming from fresh air are: regular maintenance for detoxing your bloodstream, strengthened brain function, increased mental clarity, improved digestion and respiration, reduced mental fatigue, strengthened immune system, and increased serotonin levels in the brain which creates a sense of peace and well-being. Fresh air also promotes deeper and more restful sleep and has also been shown to kill bacteria and viruses. Adding more green space into your daily activities is to your advantage. It also presents the opportunity for your body to receive a healthy dose of Vitamin D.

Vitamin D and Green Spaces

When sunlight comes in direct contact with bare skin, it works in harmony with your blood cells to naturally produce vitamin D, similar to the process of plant photosynthesis. Vitamin D, also known as the sunshine vitamin, is essential to your overall health. It can help to prevent all types of diseases to include cancer, diabetes, tuberculosis, immune disorders, osteoporosis, depression, obesity, arthritis and influenza [5]. Statistics reveal that most Americans and those living in other industrialized countries are deficient in vitamin D by as much as 66% [6]. This wide-spread deficiency stems from the fact that individuals are mostly remaining indoors and are taught that sun exposure is detrimental to their health. Without direct sunlight on the skin or eating Vitamin D rich foods, like salmon, trout, mackerel, tuna, cod liver oil, or eggs, it is difficult to get all of the vitamin D you need to experience optimal health.

Getting a healthy dose of Vitamin D from sunlight is one of God's most powerful, safe, and effective methods to naturally heal the body.

God made the two great lights, the greater light to govern the day, and the lesser light to govern the night; He made the stars also. God placed them in the expanse of the heavens to give light on the earth, and to govern the day

*and the night, and to separate the light from the darkness;
and God saw that it was good.*

Genesis 1:16-18

The only real way to know if you are deficient in vitamin D is by taking a blood test. I have my blood work completed bi-annually and make a point to have my vitamin D levels checked. The test is called the 25-hydroxy D and will help you to determine what you need to do to get your number within a healthy range. In some cases, if you are very deficient, your doctor may recommend that you take a vitamin D supplement. If your number is a little low, you can easily boost it up by eating foods that contain Vitamin D or by spending as little as 15 minutes outside in the sunlight every day.

Fresh Air: A Cure for Cancer?

Research conducted by Dr. Otto Warburg, concentrating on the lack of oxygen respiration in cells and cancer, won him his first Nobel Prize in 1931 [7]. He argued that anaerobiosis (lack of life in the absence of air or oxygen) was a primary cause of cancer cell growth and that the presence of oxygen within the bloodstream prevented cancer [8]. Much of his research has been dismissed by mainstream medicine, but it was brought back to the forefront in 2007, and is now believed to hold great promise in the war on cancer [9].

Can you imagine what the health of our world would look like if we purposely took preventative measures to develop a plan to keep our blood cells healthy by oxygenating them regularly with fresh air, coupled with other healthy lifestyle changes? This small, but very significant change can improve your quality of life, equating to tremendous health benefits. Our blood cells are simply not being nourished with enough fresh air. This is based on the fact that instead of being outside in green spaces, more, and more Americans are remaining indoors.

The Dangers of Being Surrounded by Enclosed Spaces

To give you an idea of just how many individuals are staying indoors in comparison to spending time outside, the average American spends 90%

of their time inside enclosed buildings and vehicles, leaving our blood cells with a mere 10% exposure to fresh air [10]. That's an overwhelming amount of our time being spent closed inside! God's original design involved man being one with nature and spending the majority of his lifetime outdoors. Because our physical bodies were created from the dust of the earth, we have an inborn desire to connect with being outside. This is by God's design. We must renew our thinking in this area to become more mindful of the fact that we are spiritually and physically connected to the earth. Prior to the Industrial Revolution, our ancestors spent most of their time working outdoors farming, hunting, gathering, and fishing. The statistics on sickness and disease were also drastically lower.

Are Indoor Spaces Making You Sick?

Remaining indoors for prolonged lengths of time exposes your blood cells to thousands of invisible toxins. Unfortunately, the typical modern home or office contains dozens of products that contain harmful chemicals. When these chemicals are inhaled, they can seriously and quickly damage your vital organs: lungs, heart, brain, liver, and kidneys. Using common cleaning agents such as liquid detergents, bleach, oven cleaner, laundry soap and degreasers creates a high probability that the products you are using contain toxic chemicals that are easily absorbed into the bloodstream. When inhaled, these toxins lodge and accumulate in your cells, muscle, tissues, and joints. There are countless eye-opening statistics revealing just how dangerous toxic inhalation is to the human body [11, 12, 13].

> *Cancer rates have continued to increase every year since 1970. Brain cancer in children is up 40% in 20 years. Toxic chemicals are largely to blame.*
>
> *New York Times*

An average of 148 toxic chemicals reside in our bodies.
And those were only the ones that have been tested.
The National Report on
Human Exposure to
Environmental Chemicals

The toxic chemicals in household cleaners are three times
more likely to cause cancer than air pollution.
Environmental Protection Agency (EPA)

In order to counter these statistics, part of the solution is to eliminate chemical-based products found within home, office, school, and hospital settings. About 10 years ago, I made the decision to rid my home of toxic cleaners and switched to natural cleaning alternatives. By incorporating this key and cleaning up my home environment, I was no longer subjecting my bloodstream to toxic chemical agents. By doing this, I gave my body ample time to detox and it began to heal itself. Have you ever noticed that whenever you clean your home with agents like bleach or oven cleaner, the area must be well ventilated? If you take the time to read the fine print on common cleaning products, there are several warnings printed on the bottles or packaging because manufactures are aware of the severe damage these chemicals can have on your health when you inhale them.

Sick Building Syndrome (SBS)

The term Sick Building Syndrome or (SBS) is used to describe situations where building occupants experience acute health and uncomfortable effects that appear to be linked to time spent in a building, but no specific illness or cause can be identified. The complaints may be localized in a particular room or zone, or may be widespread throughout the building. The concentration of indoor pollutants found in schools, hospitals, homes, or building environments is 2-5 times higher than the outdoor concentration of outdoor pollutants. Those affected by SBS complain of symptoms associated with acute discomfort, such as headaches, eye, nose, or throat irritation, dry cough, and dry, or itchy skin, dizziness, and nausea, difficulty in concentrating, fatigue, and sensitivity to odors [14].

The cause of the symptoms is usually not known, and most of the individuals report relief soon after leaving the building. When routinely enclosed inside of a building, the body is deprived of fresh air to properly oxygenate blood cells. Enclosed spaces subject the body to poor ventilation, synthetic materials, chemical pollutants from cleaners, toxins from heating and air conditioning units, airborne particles from dust, carpet fibers or fungal spores and when inhaled they release invisible toxins into your system, contaminating the bloodstream. The EPA has deemed poor indoor air quality as one of the top five health hazards of our generation [15].

> *Subjecting the body to enclosed spaces for prolonged periods of time, is like setting up camp in an invisible war zone; surrounded by a stealthy and unseen enemy ready to invade and attack your bloodstream with hundreds of dangerously toxic poisons.*

Research conducted by William J. Fisk and Arthur H. Rosenfield of the Lawrence Berkley Laboratory in Berkley California, revealed that when the rate of outdoor air supply (ventilation rate) is increased, the indoor air concentrations of many pollutants emitted from sources inside the building are reduced. Ventilation rate changes in U.S. offices, improved work performance by 10% and decreased SBS symptoms experienced by 12 to 16 million workers, as well as reduced 7 to 10 million days of avoided work absences. The associated total annual economic benefit ranges from $9 billion to $14 billion [16]. Not only are adults being affected by poor indoor air quality, children are no exception. Children are even more susceptible to the effects of contaminated air because they breathe in more oxygen relative to their body weight than adults. Statistics from the Centers for Disease Control and Prevention highlight the prevalence of asthma in the United States, increasing from 3.1% in 1980 to 5.5% in 1996 and 7.3% in 2001 to 8.4% in 2010, with children showing a higher rate at 9.5% in comparison to adults at 7.7% [17]. This relatively high growth rate stems from indoor and environmental toxins, presenting a major concern for health experts. In addition to

SBS, other illnesses associated with indoor toxins include: nervous system damage, reproductive challenges, auto immune disorders, blood diseases, endocrine dysfunction, chronic headaches, irritability, and visual disorders [18]. This list of illnesses is not exhaustive and can be traced back to toxins found in the bloodstream.

Toxins Are in Found in Every Day Products

Currently, the United States follows the Toxic Substances Control Act of 1976. The purpose of this act is to protect individuals from "unreasonable risk of injury to health and the environment" by regulating the safe manufacturing of chemicals products [19]. The sale of toxic products has become an annual multi-billion-dollar business and not much oversight has been given to ensure that what is being provided to consumers is safe. The selling of dangerous chemical products is contributing to an increase in diseases and adversely impacts the environment. When individuals seek to pursue the gain of wealth over the value of humanity and our environment, it is a definite concoction for disaster.

> *Certainly, the love of money is the root of all kinds of evil. Some people who have set their hearts on getting rich have wandered away from the Christian faith and have caused themselves a lot of grief.*
>
> *I Timothy 6:10*

To help you identify the source of indoor toxins, I've provided a basic reference list based upon EPA findings that will help you to begin clearing the air so to speak [20]. The list shows common items containing potentially hazardous ingredients that might be found in your home, office, childcare center, garage, basement, or other storage space. At the end of this chapter, I'll refer you to some safe and effective alternatives.

Cleaning Products

- Laundry & dish soap
- Toilet cleaners
- Wood, metal cleaners & polishes

- Drain cleaners
- Tub, tile, shower cleaners
- Bleach (laundry)
- Pool chemicals
- Oven cleaners
- Aerosol air freshener spray

Indoor Pesticides

- Ant sprays and baits
- Flea repellents & shampoos
- Bug sprays

- Household insecticides
- Moth repellents
- Mouse and rat poisons & baits

Lawn & Garden Products

- Herbicides
- Insecticides
- Fungicides/wood preservatives

- Artificial fertilizers

Automotive Products

- Motor oil
- Fuel additives
- Carburetor & fuel injection cleaners
- Air conditioning refrigerants
- Starter fluids
- Automotive batteries
- Transmission and brake fluid
- Antifreeze

Workshop/ Painting Supplies

- Adhesives and glues
- Furniture strippers
- Oil or enamel base paint
- Stains and finishes
- Paint thinners & turpentine
- Paint strippers & removers
- Photographic chemicals
- Fixatives & other solvents
- Building materials

Other Flammable Products

- Propane tanks and other compressed gas cylinders
- Kerosene
- Home heating oil
- Diesel fuel
- Gas/oil mix
- Lighter fluid
- Candles (Lead based)

Miscellaneous

- Cigarette and cigar smoke
- Plug-in oil air/room fresheners
- Hanging car air fresheners
- Plastic shower curtains and liners
- Mercury thermostats
- Fluorescent light bulbs
- Driveway sealer
- Air conditioning refrigerants
- Pet/cat litter

We are all exposed to small or larger doses of indoor and external poisons depending on your lifestyle and what region of the country you may live or work in. Toxins cannot be avoided. A wealth of information exists about the negative consequences stemming from inhaling toxic products, but having the information is not enough. Counter measures such as getting out into the fresh air and removing toxic products from your home are necessary to guard your health from these effects. Another factor contributing to the high statistics associated with being in closed spaces can be attributed to our technological advancement.

Technology and Unhealthy Lifestyle Habits

Just about every home has one or more flat screen televisions, video game systems, iPads, computers, laptops, or digital devices. I must admit that while all of these inventions are wonderful, technology has become somewhat of a stumbling block towards living healthier. Instead of going outside, teens, youth, and even adults are choosing to stay indoors, deeply immersed in Reality TV, engaged in social media or playing video games over the internet. Coupled with this, is the fact that indoor activities almost always include some form of eating unhealthy processed food such as chips, soda, sugary sweets or microwave meals. Our present and future generations are getting less exercise, less air and are becoming increasingly unhealthier. Local parks that were once filled with children, youth, and parents are becoming emptier and emptier.

In a report entitled, "Too Fat to Fight," a group of retired senior military leaders issued a warning to Congress stating that at least nine million 17 to 24-year-olds in the United States are not getting enough exercise and are too overweight to serve in the military. That equates to 27 percent of all young adults [21]. It is alarming to know that obesity rates among children and young adults have increased so dramatically that they not only threaten the overall health of America, but also weaken the strength of our military and compromises our national security.

> *Healthy citizens are the greatest asset any country can have.*
>
> *Winston Churchill*

You Must Get Up and Out, It's Time to Move...Exercise, Exercise, Exercise

One of the most important aspects of exercising is to adopt a variety of activities that are unique to you. These activities must prove to be simple, fun, enjoyable, and rewarding. Exercising outdoors boosts your health even more. When exercise is practiced on a regular basis it improves your chances of living longer and healthier, helps prevent bone loss or osteoporosis, reduces the risk of heart disease and diabetes, lowers blood pressure, relieves symptoms associated with depression, improves sleep, prevents weight gain, enhances cognitive abilities and improves heart, lung, and muscle fitness. If you are living a sedentary lifestyle, it can become costly both physically and financially.

Despite all of the excellent health benefits associated with exercise, only about 30% of individuals regularly exercise. During the past 20 years, inactivity has attributed to a dramatic increase in obesity in the United States and rates continue to rise. More than one-third of American adults (34.9%) and approximately 17% (or 12.7 million) of children and adolescents ages 2-19 are obese, resulting in a 52% overall obesity rate [22]. Physical inactivity leaves millions of individuals vulnerable to experiencing heart attacks, strokes, and depression. The potential savings if all inactive American adults became physically active in the year 2000 was $76.6 billion dollars. This figure has more than doubled in 2016 [23].

We must begin making wiser choices that are beneficial to our physical health and the financial health of our nation. Making poor choices has resulted in soaring statistics and excessive spending towards health care that could have easily been prevented by routine exercise. We were created to be physically agile beings and regular exercise is one of the best things that you can do to take care of yourself. If you're just beginning to exercise, remember to be patient with yourself and start out slow. As little as 20 minutes of outdoor exercise such as brisk walking three times a week in green space is a great place to start. If you need a little motivation to help you get started, find a fitness trainer in your area, partner with a friend or your church to help you to reach your health goals. The beginning of any journey always begins with one step. Take the first step by choosing to make a sedentary lifestyle a thing of the past. Not only will God be pleased with your efforts, your body will thank you for it too. Before closing out this chapter, I want to share one final word about an unseen toxic threat that may be resting right under your very nose.

Inhalation and Mercury Fillings

Do you or someone that you know have amalgam or "silver fillings" in your teeth? Did you know that these fillings are comprised of 50% mercury, a highly toxic chemical compound? Because fillings are located in the cavity of your mouth, millions of individuals are exposed to inhaling toxic vapors [24, 25].

> *Mercury is highly toxic and harmful to health. Approximately 80% of inhaled mercury vapor is absorbed in the blood through the lungs, causing damages to lungs, kidneys, and the nervous, digestive, respiratory, and immune systems. Health effects from excessive mercury exposure include tremors, impaired vision and hearing, paralysis, insomnia, emotional instability, developmental*

*deficits during fetal development, and attention deficit
and developmental delays during childhood.*
                      World Health Organization (WHO)

*Dental amalgam contains elemental mercury. It releases
low levels of mercury in the form of a vapor that can be
inhaled and absorbed by the lungs. High levels of mercury
vapor exposure are associated with adverse effects in the
brain and the kidneys.*
                      Food & Drug Administration (FDA)

Mercury can cause irreparable damage to the body. Many individuals are simply not aware of the dangers associated with the seemingly harmless practice of obtaining filings. Dental care for most children living in the United States begins as soon as the first tooth appears. Mercury fillings in the mouth of children present even more dangers because they are still developing and growing. From our youth, we have been told that fillings are designed to preserve the health of our teeth. While trying to protect our teeth, mercury is inhaled into the bloodstream, and we become subject to heavy metal poisoning. This toxic bloodstream circulates throughout the entire body touching the lungs, heart, kidneys, and brain. In response to the negative side-effects associated with mercury, many dentists are beginning to use safe, mercy-free fillings.

*The adage, "What you don't know can't hurt you," could
not be farther from the truth. This is a great web of
deception. Ultimately, what you don't know can hurt or
kill you and the price of ignorance becomes very high.*

Alternative Solution to Mercury Fillings

A new wave of holistic dentists is forming in America. These men and women are trained and focus on how dental care impacts your overall health. This is in contrast to conventional dentists who mainly focus on treating the teeth only. Holistic Dentistry, also known as Biological Dentistry or Alternative Dentistry, incorporates various holistic therapies

49

such as diet, lifestyle habits and may be combined with traditional methods to prevent and treat dental diseases [26].

If you do have mercury fillings, you can seek out a holistic dentist in your area to have them replaced with safe fillings or composites. It's important to note that improper removal of mercury fillings can cause serious damage to your vital organs and release more toxic mercury into your bloodstream. Before allowing any dentist to perform this procedure, ensure that you thoroughly research their working history, as well as their success rate with removing silver filings. One of the best things that you can do is to become educated about the subject of holistic dental care. In his book, *Whole Body Dentistry, A Complete Guide to Understanding the Impact of Dentistry on Total Health*, DDS, Mark A. Breiner, shares invaluable information about the paradigm taking place between conventional dentistry and holistic dentistry. Dr. Breiner is an expert in this subject and discusses oral mercury poisoning, the connection between mercury and Alzheimer's disease, and how mercury is affecting our children. This is one book that I believe needs to be read by anyone who is serious about taking their health to the next level. You can purchase this book through Amazon.com or at your local bookstore.

Breathing and Deepening Your Consciousness

The purpose of key number one, *Supplying Your Body with Fresh Air Through Exercise and Healthy Lifestyle Habits*, is to heighten and deepen your awareness of the dangers associated with inhaling toxic substances and how they impact your health. The intent for sharing this information is not to cause you to become stressful about the overwhelming prevalence of toxins that do exist, but it is to challenge you to begin thinking critically about what is impacting your health, as well equip you with essential tools to combat this silent threat.

> *God has not given us the spirit of fear, but of power, love, and a sound mind.*
>
> *2 Timothy 1:7*

God reminds us that when we receive wisdom that in all of our getting, we must also have an understanding (Prov. 4:5). We must understand that although we live in a world that is highly toxic, there are keys to counter these toxins. In this era, God is empowering His people with wisdom, knowledge, and understanding to rise up and serve as personal health guardians to protect their divine health.

> *Jesus said to them, "Surely you will quote this proverb to me: Physician, heal yourself!"*
>
> *Luke 4:23a*

This sound piece of advice from Jesus lets us know that we must take personal action, to bring about healing and wholeness in our own lives on spiritual and physical levels. God's will is for Christians to live healthy abundant lives, and we have a very important role to play in our physical healing, for faith without works is dead.

Let's Get Back to the Beginning

When God created Adam and Eve, He placed them in the Garden of Eden, in wide-open spaces to interact with nature and to experience the healing benefits of creation. In all of His infinite wisdom, God placed the sun in just the right position, not too close or too far away, to provide the earth and His children with an adequate supply of sunshine. He skillfully designed the outdoor environment with the precise levels of oxygen that we would need to sustain the earth and to keep us healthy. Key number one, getting out into the fresh air, was the first stepping-stone that God provided to us in our wellness plan. As God's people, we must return to this most essential, natural, and basic key to maintain our health. This was and still is God's original design.

> *Now the Lord God had planted a garden in the east, in Eden, and there he put the man he had formed. The Lord God made all kinds of trees grow out of the ground—trees that were pleasing to the eye and good for food. In the middle of the garden were the tree of life and the tree of the knowledge of good and evil.*
>
> *Genesis 2:8-9*

Key # 1 - Supply Your Body with Fresh Air
Through Exercise and Healthy Lifestyle Habits

Healthy Ways to Rock Your World Naturally with Fresh Air

- Make a habit of opening all of the windows in your home regularly, if not daily to allow fresh air to circulate through all of the rooms in your house.

- Use ceiling fans or circulating fans instead of air conditioning units to keep your home ventilated and cool.

- Fill your office or home with living plants. During photosynthesis, plants release an abundance of oxygen into the atmosphere.

- Practice focused breathing during your walks for at least 15-30 minutes daily 5 times a week. Be sure to concentrate on your breathing i.e. inhaling deeply through your nose and exhaling completely through your mouth. If walking during the colder months, be sure to wear layers to stay warm. This is an invigorating way to jumpstart your day.

- Establish an exercise routine outside 4-5 times weekly. Consider splitting your exercise routine 50/50 i.e. workout half indoors and half outdoors. If you need a partner to help you stick to your workout commitment, connect with someone from your church or in your community to stay accountable.

- Practice deep breathing exercises 5 times a week for at least 15 minutes near an open window, door, or outside.

- When working indoors, take your breaks outside instead of remaining inside.

- If within reasonable distance, opt to walk or ride your bike to work. Not only is this great for your health, it also reduces the emissions that are released into the environment by vehicle fumes and exhaust.

- Get off of the couch and out into the great outdoors often by visiting local parks, hiking trails or beaches.

- Drive with the windows down and/or sunroof open in your car especially while driving through green spaces.

- If you have mercury fillings, seek out a holistic dentist to have them safely removed.

- Opt for using all natural air fresheners such as soy based and beeswax candles and essential oils. The chemicals found in most candles, plug-in air fresheners and sprays contain large amounts of carcinogenic (cancer-causing) substances.

- Go green with environmentally safe cleaning products. You can purchase safe cleaning products from Seventh Generation at www.seventhgeneration.com or you can easily make your own by using basic items found in your kitchen such as baking soda, lemons, vinegar, or distilled water. Homemade products are safe and highly effective and will make your home or office amazingly clean for pennies on the dollar.

- Recipe for bathtub and sink scrub. In a bowl, make a paste with baking soda, a squirt of Seventh Generation Natural Dish Liquid and a squeeze of lemon. Dip your cloth or sponge into paste and scrub. Allow the paste to sit for 10-15 minutes for hard to remove grime. Rinse when complete.

- Recipe for mirror and glass cleaner. Mix 2 teaspoons of vinegar and 1 quart of water in a reusable spray bottle. Spray the mixture on mirror or glass, and wipe clean with an old cotton cloth.

- Recipe for floor cleaner. Combine 1/4 cup of Seventh Generation natural dish liquid, 1/2 cup of white vinegar or lemon juice in 2 gallons of warm water in a sink or large bucket. You can use this on any floor, unless the manufacturer has specified to avoid all detergents.

- If you have yard space, consider investing in a clothes line to dry your clothes. By drying your clothes outside, you'll decrease the amount of environmental toxins released from the dryer and you'll also save on your energy bills.

- Have you ever noticed the strong smell that permeates the atmosphere when you take a vinyl shower curtain or liner out of the package? That is the smell of hundreds of toxic chemicals. Protect you and your family by replacing toxic vinyl shower curtains and liners with cloth shower curtains and liners.

- Rid your home of products that contain hazardous chemicals and replace them with safe, effective, and natural alternatives. For alternative choices visit http://www.osha.gov and http://www2.epa.gov/saferchoice.

Key # 2

Love, Protect & Nurture Your Skin

[Absorption / assimilate; to take in or include as part of oneself]

Do you not know that your body is the temple of the living God?

I Corinthians 3:16a

What spirit is so empty and blind, that it cannot recognize the fact that the foot is more noble than the shoe, and skin more beautiful than the garment with which it is clothed?
Michelangelo

Chapter 3

Learn to Love the Skin That You're In

T he human body is an extraordinary beautiful masterpiece composed of 700 muscles, 206 bones, 30 trillion cells, 25 miles of blood vessels, and about 5 liters of blood [1]. Our internal framework of organs function in seamless fashion to keep us aligned and balanced. The human anatomy is nothing short of miraculous.

I will praise You, for I am fearfully made; marvelous are Your works, and my soul knows very well.
Psalms 139:14

Often shrouded by the latest fashion trends, perfumes, colognes, makeup, and sprays, we rarely hear about the importance of caring for the health of the skin, but rather our focus is drawn towards the external adornment of the body. Bombarded by one new advertisement after the other, crowds are mesmerized by commercials featuring a gorgeous woman, an attractive man or an adorable baby taking center stage as they showcase the latest vogue in modern makeup, designer fragrance or baby product to help keep your baby smelling "baby fresh." Behind all of the glossy advertisements, a true endangerment to your health exists involving skin absorption. In this chapter, you'll discover why what you are putting on your skin really does matter.

Just How Important is Your Skin?

The skin is external and is regarded as the largest organ on the human body, and covers about 20 square feet on the average size person. The skin is responsible for several vital functions. Let's take a look at what the skin does.

- It is the first line of defense against sickness and disease

- It serves as protective covering for the body

- It absorbs vital nutrients to keep the body healthy

- It holds our bodies together

- It is the passage way to our bloodstream

- It helps removes toxins from the body through our sweat glands

- It plays a vital role in manufacturing vitamin D from the sun

- It aids in regulating our body temperature

- It aids the blood in naturally healing cuts, bruises, and punctures

The proper care of our skin is essential to our health because skin absorbs up to 60% of what is placed on it [2]. Most of what we put on our skin is toxic, especially personal care products.

So...What's the Problem with Personal Care Products?

You know the drill, your morning routine. Just about everyone has one. Yours may look a little something like this. You hear the alarm go off and you tap the snooze button on your smartphone for about third time hoping to squeeze in a few more minutes of sleep just before starting the day. You get up out of bed, brush your teeth, jump in the shower, use your favorite body wash, fix your hair with gel and hairspray, put on your makeup, get dressed and put on your favorite fragrance. You spend your morning devotion time with God. You're out the door in just enough time to stop by Dunkin Donuts to pick up a few breakfast items along with your favorite coffee before heading in to the office. It seems like nothing out of the ordinary and you feel fine right? Before leaving your house, what you don't realize is that you have unknowingly overloaded your body with hundreds of poisonous toxins from the products that you innocently used.

On average, individuals use about ten personal care products daily, containing hundreds of harmful ingredients. These products usually consist of items like hair gel, body lotion, perfume, baby powder, bar soap, body wash, hair dyes, toothpaste, nail polish, makeup, and shampoo. Although these products are sold over the counter, it does not mean they are safe. The FDA is not required by law to test the safety of products that are being sold [3, 4].

> *"...A cosmetic manufacturer may use almost any raw material as a cosmetic ingredient and market the product without an approval from FDA. The FDA does no systematic reviews of safety, instead authorizing the cosmetics industry to self-police ingredient safety through its Cosmetics Ingredient Review panel."*
> *Office of Cosmetics and Colors,*
> *Food and Drug Administration*

One would expect those in authority to ensure that policies in place not only classify products, but also regulate their safety to human health. Disappointingly, this is not the case.

What's Actually In My Personal Care Products?

Because the FDA does not conduct routine safety reviews on personal care product ingredients, just about anything is acceptable under the current law. If the manufacturer of a product determines that a toxic chemical ingredient is necessary for use and is relatively safe permitted by their standards, it is permissible under the existing FDA regulation. The FDA has left the safety review of ingredients as the sole responsibility of the Cosmetic Ingredients Review panel although thousands of products are not considered cosmetics such as cologne, toothpaste, soap, shaving cream, deodorant, mouthwash, feminine products, body wash etc. and are left at the discretion of the manufacturer for safety.

Not having an approved standard in place for manufacturers to verify the safety of toxic chemicals used in personal care products continues to pose a serious health threat to consumers. Below are some of the most common chemical substances that are hazardous to our health.

- Dibutyl phthalate: this chemical is used in hair spray and nail care products. It has been shown to disrupt the endocrine system and is toxic to the reproductive system and hinders the development of organs in unborn children [5].

- Formaldehyde: is listed as a known carcinogen with the National Toxicology Program (NTP) and is found in nail polishes, nail hardeners, eyelash glues, hair gels, soaps, makeup, shampoos, lotions, and deodorants [6].

- Triclosan: is used in antibacterial cleaners, toothpaste, and household products. It has been shown to cause sexual dysfunction, infertility, and birth defects. This chemical has also been linked to heart problems, cancer of the liver, immune system disorders, brain hemorrhaging and paralysis [7].

- Parabens: are used in food, skin moisturizers, cosmetics, and pharmaceuticals. They have been shown to adversely affect the male reproductive system and negatively impair functions of the spleen, liver, kidney, and adrenal gland. Ongoing research is being conducted to determine the correlation between the use of parabens in deodorant and breast cancer [8].

The NTP prepares the Report on Carcinogens (RoC) on behalf of the Secretary of Health and Human Services. The RoC is a congressionally mandated, science-based, public health report that identifies agents, substances, mixtures, or exposures (collectively called "substances") in our environment that may potentially put people in the United States at increased risk for cancer [9]. You can visit their web site to review the report, as well as become further educated on the thousands of other dangerously toxic chemicals found in personal care products at http://ntp.niehs.nih.gov/pubhealth/roc/index.html.

Wake Up Before It's Too Late

There is an interesting 19th century science experiment that I learned about in college that you may or may not be familiar with. Researchers discovered that when they placed a frog in a pot of boiling water, the frog quickly jumped out. On the other hand, when they put a frog in cold water and slightly increased the heat of the water to boiling point, the frog did not jump out, but just sat there and boiled to death [10]. The hypothesis infers that because the change in temperature is so gradual, the frog does not realize that it's slowly boiling to death. While the results of the experiment are rather drastic, it is an excellent metaphor concerning toxins and skin absorption. Initially, individuals don't feel the effects of the toxic environment that is gradually being formed in their bloodstream. They don't feel any different. Everything appears to be fine externally, but an internal war is raging. The bloodstream is fighting extremely hard to stay healthy by expelling harmful toxins.

Skin Absorption and the Internal War

The chief function of white blood cells in the body's immune system is to protect the body against harmful substances stemming from toxins, infection, bacteria, and cancerous cells. The principal role of red blood cells is to transport oxygen to our vital organs to keep them healthy and operating at peak performance. If the bloodstream is overflowing with toxins, and not cleansed regularly, how can anyone avoid contracting some form of illness? The answer is you cannot.

Barraged with toxins from the use of everyday personal care products, the bloodstream becomes inundated with pollutants. The presence of toxins causes the white blood cells to respond by fighting them off, however, too many toxins weaken and compromise the immune system. Instead of providing protection for the body, white blood cells are forced into survival mode, causing confusion and malfunction within the body. The white blood cells cannot distinguish between toxins, good or bad bacteria or infections and begin attacking them all to include healthy red blood cells. When healthy cells begin to attack themselves, this is known as an autoimmune disorder. If this toxic cycle continues, the battle will be lost to one or more of the innumerable health disorders we see plaguing our world today in the form of arthritis, Irritable Bowel Syndrome, asthma, eczema, chronic inflammation, ADD/ADHD, psychological disorders, allergies, and various cancers.

Autoimmune Disorders Are On the Rise

The National Institute of Health reports that there are over 80 different types of autoimmune disorders [11]. The latest research reveals that 8% of the population, 78% of whom are women, has been diagnosed with an autoimmune disorder. Autoimmune disorders are among the top 10 most common causes of death for people younger than 64 years old [12]. Because autoimmune diseases debilitate the function of red blood cells, the heart, brain, eyes, joints, lungs, kidneys, glands, nerves, muscles, skin, and digestive tract do not receive adequate supplies of oxygen-rich nutrients to stay healthy. The most common autoimmune diseases are:

- Graves Disease
- Rheumatoid Arthritis
- Hashimoto's Thyroiditis
- Type I Diabetes
- Pernicious Anemia
- Multiple Sclerosis
- Ulcerative Colitis
- Systemic Lupus

- Celiac disease
- Chron's disease
- Fibromyalgia
- Alopecia
- Juvenile Arthritis
- Lyme disease chronic
- Systemic Lupus
- Endometriosis

The statistics are higher for women due to the fact that women may be exposed to absorbing more toxic chemicals through their skin than men, specifically in the areas of designer fragrances, cleaning products, hair sprays, nail polish, hair coloring and makeup applications. If you glance through any popular women's magazine, you will discover that most of the advertisements promote products that must be applied to the skin; the latest must have eye shadows, hair coloring, lotions, mascaras, creams, lip sticks, eye liners and perfumes. The cost of looking and smelling good comes with too high of a price that is robbing us of our divine health.

A Special Word on Beauty

God has such a different view on what He considers to be beautiful. His ways and His thoughts are certainly not like ours. Have you ever met someone who is considered to be strikingly handsome or very beautiful and after talking or spending time with him or her, you discovered that they had the worst attitude? Despite being physically attractive, their personality made them unattractive and unpleasant to be around. When king Saul defied God, He provided Samuel with His perspective on outer appearances:

But the LORD said to Samuel, "Do not consider his appearance or his height, for I have rejected him. The LORD does not look at the things man looks at. Man looks at the outward appearance, but the LORD looks at the heart."

I Samuel 16:7

I believe that God wants us to look our very best, but more importantly, He is more concerned that our hearts are right before Him. We need to ask ourselves: Am I obeying God in word, thought, and deed? Am I kind and loving towards humanity? Are my actions pleasing to God? When you genuinely commit to work on developing your personal walk with God, there is a radiant glow that comes out of your relationship with Him. There is a special joy that God fills you with, known as the oil of joy. David said it best, "You will show me the path of life. In Your presence, there is fullness of joy, at Your right hand there are pleasures forevermore," (Psalms 16:11). This special infilling will cause you to reflect and walk in the fruit of the spirit as described in Galatians 5:22-26:

But the fruit of the [Holy] Spirit [the work which His presence within accomplishes] is love, joy (gladness), peace, patience (an even temper, forbearance), kindness, goodness (benevolence), faithfulness, gentleness (meekness, humility), self-control (self-restraint, continence). Against such things there is no law [that can bring a charge].

God's power working on the inside of you will attract the attention of others, opening the door of invitation to introduce them to a personal relationship with Jesus Christ. Everyday millions of bold, creative, and eye-catching glossy advertisements resonate with the message that individuals can obtain radiant and flawless beauty with just a few applications of the newest beauty creation. Men and women everywhere strive to enhance their natural beauty, without realizing that what is being absorbed through their skin is nothing less than dangerous and deadly. In a world that is focused on outer beauty, let us be ever mindful of what God's says about being beautiful. Know that you are fearfully and wonderfully made and are absolutely beautiful in His sight! Beauty begins on the inside.

It's Time to Begin Thinking Critically

While walking through the mall one day, I was suddenly stopped in my tracks by what I saw. I came across a nail salon that was filled with nail technicians and clientele. All of the nail technicians were wearing facial masks and gloves. Not that I have not ever seen this before, but this time, the facial masks stood out to me even more on that particular day.

Have you ever taken the time to question why nail technicians wear facial masks and gloves all day long when providing their clients with manicures and pedicures? These protective coverings must be worn to prevent inhaling and absorbing toxic chemicals. Nail technicians are in this type of working atmosphere for long periods of time and need to be protected for health reasons. Clients visit these establishments quite often, if not weekly, for one to two hours at a time and are not protected with any type of protective covering. Remember the frog scenario? Inhaling and absorbing chemical toxins even if only for a few hours, may seem harmless, but when practiced over extended periods of time, health complications will arise. Men and women leave these establishments not only inhaling, but have also absorbed hundreds of chemicals into their bloodstream through nail polish, nail gels and other bodily applications. What I saw made me wonder how many people are suffering from some type of physical illness stemming from repeated trips to the nail salon.

Why Are Chemical Laced Products Allowed to Be Sold?

The distribution and selling of personal care products is big business. In 2010, Americans spent $33.3 billion on cosmetics and other beauty products, up 6% from 2009 [13]. As stated in the FDA regulation, the onus lies with the manufacturer to ensure the safety of products being sold. If the FDA intervened and held manufactures to a higher level of accountability the government, manufactures, and corporations would suffer a great financial loss. It is paradoxical that Americans are spending billions of dollars on personal care products annually and at the same time, we are spending billions of dollars annually on treating illnesses. The connection between these two industries is undeniable. The good news is that it doesn't have to remain this way.

Use Products that Are Safe for Your Skin

Just as there are countless products on the market that are detrimental to our health, there are thousands of alternatives available that provide an abundance of nourishment and healing to your skin. One industry leader that champions the use of safe, non-toxic personal care products is the Environmental Working Group (EWG). As a result of their diligent efforts, they have spearheaded a movement known as Skin Deep™.

> *Through Skin Deep™, we [EWG] put the power of information in consumers' hands. When you know what's in the products you bring into your home and how those chemicals may affect your health and the environment, you can make informed purchasing decisions — and help transform the marketplace. At the same time, we advocate responsible corporate and governmental policies to protect the most vulnerable among us.*
>
> *Environmental Working Group*

To further heighten consumer awareness, the EWG created an outstanding free app for Skin Deep™ called Healthy Living. The Healthy Living app allows you to scan the bar codes of personal care products that will reveal whether the products are toxic or non-toxic. The app allows you to look up a product, research ingredients, search a company by name and find safer alternatives. The safety for each product is based on a rating scale of 0 to 10, with the lower end of the scale ranging from safe 0-2, moderate 3-6 and hazardous from 7-10.

I highly recommend this app and have made it a part of my regular shopping experience. I am continually taken back when I discover that products that I thought were safe are in fact not. It has been a real eye-opener for me. I share this with you to emphasize the fact that just because a product carries the words "organic" or "natural" does not necessarily mean that they are safe to use. In the United States, the laws governing the use of the terms organic and natural are loosely defined. For instance, the product could consist of only one or two organic ingredients and still carry the title "organic," while the other 20-30 substances are extremely toxic. Natural simply refers to what was used to make the product and is solely deemed to be "natural" by the chemist or scientist creating the product. By the time the product is completed, the natural source is so processed that it is no longer in its natural state, however, by law it can still be labeled "natural" [14]. The term natural is merely used as a marketing strategy to get consumers to buy their product because people believe that it is safer. In some countries, the term "natural" is enforced and well-defined, while in the United States it has no meaning.

I encourage you to download the Healthy Living app on your digital device to help you to consistently practice *Loving, Nurturing, and Protecting Your Skin*. Also, be sure to visit EWG's web site at http://www.ewg.org to find out how you can become a part of the Skin Deep™ movement. A good rule of thumb to follow is the fewer the ingredients a product contains, the safer it usually is. Maintaining the health of your skin is not just about what you put on it, but it also includes what you put into our body. Invisible toxins surround us, they are in our air and food, so what you eat also contributes to having healthy, clear, glowing skin. The Healthy Living app also rates over 80,000 foods to help you understand what you are putting into your body. The importance of clean eating will be shared in the upcoming chapters.

Change the Law by Letting Your Voice Be Heard

As with any major change involving national laws or regulations, change begins by changing the law itself. In March 2015, bill S.725, Alan Reinstein and Trevor Schaefer Toxic Chemical Protection Act, was introduced by Senator Barbra Boxer (D-CA) to amend the current Toxic Substance Control Act of 1976 [15]. The bill asks for the following requirement to be implemented: "Reform of this Act shall be administered to protect the health of children, pregnant women, the elderly, workers, consumers, the general public and the environment from the risks of harmful exposures to chemical substances and mixtures." The bill also requests additional actions, however this is the top area of interest.

At the moment, S.725 is still in the initial stages and at the time of writing this book, 5 of the 50 United States representatives support this bill. No major actions have taken place, but it is promising to see the leadership of our nation acknowledging the gravity of the issue. Seeking out viable solutions to establish a safety standard for toxic ingredients being used in personal care products is long overdue. Bill S.725 also requests that animals not be used to test toxic chemical ingredients. "Funding research and validation studies to reduce, refine, and replace the use of animal tests in accordance with this subsection." Currently, the Toxic Substance Control Act of 1976 permits animal testing for toxic chemical products. While animal testing still takes place in America, the European Union banned the use of animal testing on all personal care products in 2004. Even more recently, in 2013, European regulators declared a ban on the import and sale of cosmetics containing ingredients tested on animals and pledged their efforts to push other parts of the world to accept alternatives [16].

Animal testing of any sort is not necessary, and as a part of God's creation animals should be treated humanely. America desperately needs change to take place concerning the current regulations to preserve human health, and at the same time we must ensure the protection and safety of all animals. There is an adage that says, "the squeaky wheel gets the oil." If enough voices are heard to persistently urge US representatives to amend the current Toxic Substance Act to promote an industry standard that mandates the use of safe toxic-free ingredients without animal testing it would prove to be a monumental step towards change for the betterment of all.

As a nation, we have a moral responsibility to become actively engaged in issues that adversely affect our society. In essence, negative circumstances can serve as the catalyst to foster positive changes within our world through prayer and action. The bible reminds us that God wants us to pray for earthly kings, presidents, governors, and all those in authority that we may lead quiet and peaceable lives in all godliness and honesty. God can and does use our prayers to intervene on behalf of our nation so that those in authority will be saved and eventually come to know the truth about God's saving grace.

First of all, then, I admonish and urge that petitions, prayers, intercessions, and thanksgivings be offered on behalf of all men, for kings and all who are in positions of authority or high responsibility, that [outwardly] we may pass a quiet and undisturbed life [and inwardly] a peaceable one in all godliness and reverence and seriousness in every way. For such [praying] is good and right, and [it is] pleasing and acceptable to God our Savior, who wishes all men to be saved and [increasingly] to perceive and recognize and discern and know precisely and correctly the [divine] Truth.

1 Timothy 2:1-4

Through united efforts, we can become involved to help implement favorable laws for our nation. Throughout the bible, God used judges, priests, prophets and everyday ordinary people to bring about social justice to the poor, widows, children, and the outcasts of society. If you have never written to your representatives before, here's your opportunity to be a part of the change you want to see. You can view bill S.725 in its entirety by visiting http://www.congress.gov. Find the search box at the top of the page and type in the bill number S.725. Be sure to submit your comments and let your voice be heard about your desire to see this bill changed and implemented as a law.

Being a Good Steward of Your Temple

Your skin is the outer covering of your temple and it needs proper care and attention to achieve a healthier lifestyle. We can't overlook the fact that personal care products are a huge part of our lives. Though change to remove dangerous toxins from these products is on the horizon, it will take time for industry standards and laws to come into fruition. In the meantime, you can take action on a personal level by committing to use products that are not detrimental to your overall health. By eliminating toxic personal care products, you will give your body time to detox, heal, repair, and recover. The impact on your health is too high of a price to pay to not use this key. By using this key, to *Love, Protect, and Nurture Your Skin*, you will unlock amazing health benefits. Your health will soar to new heights and you can experience the energy and vitality you've been longing for. Because the skin plays such a critical role in our health, the next chapter is dedicated to third way that toxins enter the bloodstream by way of injection.

Key # 2 - Love, Protect & Nurture Your Skin

Healthy Ways to Rock Your Skin Naturally

- Clean up your world by eliminating toxic products. Download EWG's Healthy Living app on your smartphone or tablet to search for safe non-toxic alternatives to include: nail polish, cosmetics, skin care, lotions, shampoo, hair coloring, perfume, body wash, deodorant, and more.

- Allow your skin to breath. Your skin is a living organ and absorbs oxygen and releases carbon dioxide. At times, one of the best things you can do for your skin is to not apply anything to it all. Fresh air in green space is one of the best healing agents for your skin.

- Place quality filters on your bathroom showerheads and faucets. Using a quality filter will remove harmful compounds such as chlorine, copper, and other trace metals that can be absorbed into your bloodstream. To see what water filter works best for your lifestyle visit http://www.waterfiltercomparisons.com.

- Feed your skin with a healthy dose of sunshine. When sunlight comes in contact with bare skin, it produces vitamin D. Vitamin D aids in killing bacteria and fungi and naturally heals the skin. As little as 15 minutes in the sunshine every day is an excellent source of healing.

- Exercising 4-5 times weekly encourages your body to sweat. Sweating naturally rids your body of toxins that clog your pores. Taking a shower directly after working out washes off the toxins that have been released. In addition, exercise increases oxygen and blood flow within the skin and gives it a natural healthy glow.

- Locate a holistic spa or wellness center in your area that uses infrared saunas. Individuals are becoming more knowledgeable about the therapeutic healing properties associated with using infrared saunas. The radiant heat provides all of the healthy benefits of natural sunlight. This is especially beneficial during colder winter months. Infrared saunas have been shown to improve blood circulation, detox the bloodstream, strengthen the immune system and moisturize your skin.

• Write to your Congressional leader in support of bill S.725, Alan Reinstein and Trevor Schaefer Toxic Chemical Protection Act and request that the current Toxic Substances Control Act of 1976 be amended or replaced with a new law to enforce the removal of toxic substances from personal care products by visiting www.congress.gov. Type S.725 in the search bar to view the bill in its entirety.

Part II

Key # 2

Love, Protect & Nurture Your Skin

*[Injection / to drive or force a solution
or medicine etc. into the body through
the skin by or as if by syringe]*

*Do you not know that your body is the
temple of the living God?*

I Corinthians 3:16a

Unsafe injection practices are an international issue. With an estimated 16 million injections administered annually in developing and transitional countries alone, the importance of promoting safe injection practices is unprecedented.
World Health Organization

Chapter 4

What Are You Injecting Into Your World?

———————•———————

T his chapter will continue to focus on the second key to unlocking extraordinary health, *Love, Protect and Nurture Your Skin* and will discuss why you must be mindful about what is being injected into your bloodstream. Injection occurs when a sharp object (e.g., needle) punctures the skin and injects a chemical or virus directly into the bloodstream[1]. Today, individuals are participating in a wide variety of injections for tattoos, immunizations, Botox treatments, pain management, tanning, vitamin deficiency, medication, drug use and steroids. Do I believe that all injections are harmful? No, but I do believe that it is vitally important for individuals to become educated about the negative effects that some injections can have on their health. Once you receive the education, you can make an informed decision and choose what works best for you prior to injections being introduced into your bloodstream. We'll start off by taking a look at the ever-popular tattoo.

Tattoos and You

Yes, it seems that just about everyone you know has a tattoo. Tattoos can range from being simple and small to extensive and detailed. Every few years, there is a tattoo expo in my state, drawing in thousands   of people from all over the world, providing a platform for artists to showcase their most creative work. In the military, tattoos are a part   of tradition and seem to serve as a rite of passage. When I completed technical school training in the Air Force, my roommate and I were going to get tattoos together. She went through with it and I chickened out. Over the years, I've seen individuals disqualified for entry into military service or denied employment because of their tattoos. Often filled with regret, they made their decision in haste to get the tattoo and wish that had never gone through with it. Tattoos are a controversial subject for Christians. Some believe that it's okay to get a tattoo and others do not. Outside of all of our opinions, what does the bible say about tattoos? Tattoos are mentioned in the bible one time.

> *"Do not cut your bodies for the dead or put tattoo marks on yourselves. I am the LORD."*
>
> *Leviticus 19:28*

In order to get a clear understanding of this scripture, we must review the historical background of the text. The book of Leviticus is a book of laws given to priests to share how God wanted the children of Israel to live. At this particular time, God's people were surrounded by several pagan nations that served and worshiped a number of idol gods. God did not want them to be influenced by immoral practices such as worshipping the dead, sacrificing their children to idol gods or offering up food to pagan gods. In response, God told the children of Israel not to cut their bodies for the dead because the practice of making deep gashes on the face and arms and legs, in time of bereavement, was universal among pagan nations [2]. The book of I Kings provides an example of cutting the flesh when the prophet Elijah confronted the prophets of Baal about their pagan worship.

At noon Elijah began to taunt them. "Shout louder!" he said. "Surely he is a god! Perhaps he is deep in thought, or busy, or traveling. Maybe he is sleeping and must be awakened." So they shouted louder and slashed themselves with swords and spears, as was their custom, until their blood flowed. Midday passed, and they continued their frantic prophesying until the time for the evening sacrifice. But there was no response, no one answered, no one paid attention.

I Kings 18:27-29

Cutting the flesh was considered to be a mark of respect for the dead, as well as a sort of offering to the deities who presided over death and the grave. God also told them that He did not want them to print any marks on their bodies by tattooing or imprinting figures on various parts of their body because pagan nations did this in honor of an idol god.

Tattoos and Spiritual implications

While it may be unlikely that Christians today are getting tattoos to pay respect to the dead or to honor idol gods, there are other biblical principles that indicate that tattoos are inappropriate, and I'll explain why by way of the scriptures. The bible reminds us in I Corinthians 3:17 AMP, "If anyone does hurt to God's temple *or* corrupts it [with false doctrines] *or* destroys it, God will do hurt to him *and* bring him to the corruption of death *and* destroy him. For the temple of God is holy (sacred to Him) and that [temple] you [the believing church and its individual believers] are. We must realize that we are the very living, breathing sanctuaries of God, housing His very presence. Because God lives in us, He requires us to maintain and protect our temple from any and all forms of spiritual corruption and physical hurt. When tattoos are impressed upon the skin, the original design that God intended for your temple becomes damaged. Tattooing is a very painful procedure, permanently scarring and sometimes burning the flesh, bringing hurt to God's temple. From the very beginning, God made a clear distinction between pagan ways and the law of God. His desire has always been for His children to come out of and be separate from the world around us and not to blend in. Our standard of living must reflect God's values and His way of thinking. Although our times and seasons have changed, the ways of God never change.

> *So, come out from among [unbelievers], and separate (sever) yourselves from them, says the Lord, and touch not [any] unclean thing; then I will receive you kindly and treat you with favor. And I will be a Father to you, and you shall be My sons and daughters, says the Lord Almighty.*
> *2 Corinthians 6:17-18*

> *For I, the LORD, do not change; therefore you, O sons of Jacob, are not consumed.*
> *Malachi 3:6*

Tattoos and Health Implications

As the spiritual aspects of tattooing have been explored, the health concerns surrounding tattoos will be examined. Tattooing has proven to be extremely detrimental to the health of the blood. Research continually shows that a number of diseases can be transmitted due to the reuse of unclean needles. The transmission of several infectious diseases has been associated with tattooing, also known as Transfusion Transmitted Diseases (TTDs). Strong evidence shows the transmission of hepatitis B virus (HBV) infection, hepatitis C virus (HCV) infection, and syphilis from tattooing [3]. Tattooing may also transmit the Human Immunodeficiency Virus (HIV) and Acquired Human Immunodeficiency Virus (AIDS), however studies are still being conducted to validate this.

In their report entitled, Think Before You Ink: Are Tattoos Safe? The FDA, states that they have not legally approved any tattoo pigments for injection into the skin [4]. This applies to all tattoo pigments, including those used for ultraviolet (UV) and glow-in-the dark tattoos. Many pigments used in tattoo inks are industrial-grade colors suitable for office printers' ink or automobile paint. Tattoo inks may also be highly carcinogenic (cause cancer). There is ongoing research to show the correlation between cancer and the many toxins found in tattoo dyes. Several tattoo inks contain lead, mercury, iron oxide, cobalt nickel and arsenic, all of which when enter the bloodstream poison the body and effect vital organs. God always gives us laws and boundaries to protect us from unknown dangers. When the law concerning tattoos was provided, it was given with our well-being and future in mind.

> *For I know the thoughts that I have for you, says the Lord,*
> *thoughts and plans for welfare and peace and not for evil,*
> *to give you hope in your final outcome.*
>
> > *Jeremiah 29:11*

The spiritual and health implications reveal the many dangers associated with tattoos. Please understand that if you do have a tattoo, this is not to condemn you or to require you to have it removed, but to shed light on the various aspects of this practice. We must begin making conscious efforts to protect our living temples.

The Real Fountain of Youth

Collagen, Botox, and tanning injections have become a major fad in America. Thousands of men and women are trying desperately to maintain and enhance their youthful looks with these "youth serum" injections. Naturally, we must all go through different seasons in life. There are seasons when we are young and inevitably, barring accidental or premature death, there will come a time when we will age. As individuals strive to hold on to the fountain of youth, the meaning of growing older for the Christian differs in comparison to those who have no hope in Christ. The bible says that growing old comes with great wisdom and honor.

> *Gray hair is a crown of glory; it is gained by living a*
> *godly life.*
>
> > *Proverbs 16:13*

The glory of young men is their strength, gray hair the splendor of the old.

Proverbs 20:29

Much like my neighbor Jennie, at the age of 93, she is enjoying her golden years and all that comes with it. My neighborhood has adopted her as the matriarch of our community. In addition to her sons visiting her daily, someone is always checking on her to make sure that she has what she needs. Jennie always gives back by sharing her wisdom. She often gives insight about the lessons she's learned in life and how important family values, friendships, faith, and community are to her. She is a wonderful example of enjoying the golden years.

Society has conditioned us to believe that the first sight of gray hair is usually associated with getting old and is seen as something bad. I am not against coloring your hair, if it's done safely. I want to challenge you to think about why you are doing what you are doing. I mention this only because, preserving youthful looks, usually begins with dying your hair, which can lead to other treatments like injections. It is essential to our emotional health to fully accept and confidently rest in who we are in every season of life, when we are young, as well as when we age.

The media continually promotes advertisements involving beautiful young women and strong handsome young men, creating the illusion that being young is somehow better than being older. There is much more to life than possessing youthful looks. Let's face it, generally when we're in our early twenties we really don't know much of anything. We're actually just beginning to grow into adulthood and discovering how life works. In our thirties, we become more knowledgeable and display greater confidence about moving in the world. It's a time when most individuals seem to be a bit more settled. By the time we reach our forties, most of us are established in our careers and have set and accomplished many of our life goals. We have developed a greater level of understanding and maturity and flow in our lane so speak.

The greatest time of creativity in an individual's life manifests between sixty and eighty years of age. Individuals generate new ideas at a rate exceeding their younger years due to the experience gained from life lessons and because they have simply lived longer than someone who is twenty years old. Here are a few examples validating this point. At the age of ninety-six, world-renowned Evangelist Billy Graham's desire to share the hope of Christ is still as strong, if not stronger, as it was when he first started evangelizing, as a young man. In 2014, he produced a short film entitled, Heaven, which shares his thoughts about heaven and how others can make heaven their eternal home. At the age of sixty- four, in addition to her many influential literary works and notable life achievements, as a dancer, actress, and singer, Maya Angelou penned and read a poem at President Bill Clinton's Inauguration and at the age of sixty-nine and she did it again for President Barack Obama at the age of eighty [5]. Mother Teresa dedicated her life to serving the poorest populations well into her seventies. Through her devoted service, she was the catalyst for establishing centers for the blind, aged, and disabled. At the ages of fifty-eight and sixty-nine, she was summoned to Rome to receive the Nobel Peace Prize for her humanitarian work [6].

> *"By blood, I am Albanian. By citizenship, an Indian. By faith, I am a Catholic nun. As to my calling, I belong to the world. As to my heart, I belong entirely to the Heart of Jesus."*
>
> *Mother Teresa*

In the Old Testament, when Caleb came before Joshua to obtain his portion of the promised land, he told him that even though he was eighty-five years old, he was just a strong as he was when God first called them into battle.

> *"Now behold, the LORD has let me live, just as He spoke, these forty-five years, from the time that the LORD spoke this word to Moses, when Israel walked in the wilderness; and now behold, I am eighty-five years old today. I am still as strong today as I was in the day Moses sent me; as my strength was then, so my strength is now, for war and for going out and coming in. Now then, give me this hill country about which the LORD spoke on that day, for you heard on that day that Anakim were there, with great fortified cities; perhaps the LORD will be with me, and I will drive them out as the LORD has spoken." So*

> *Joshua blessed him and gave Hebron to Caleb the son of*
> *Jephunneh for an inheritance.*
>
> *Joshua 14:10-13*

Just as God had a special plan for Evangelist Billy Graham, Maya Angelou, Mother Teresa and Caleb, He has purpose for every one of us. Life can be so much greater and even more fulfilling than the earlier years that we experience. Throughout the bible, some of the greatest events recorded in history took place late in a person's life. Abraham, Sarah, Moses, and Anna are prime examples of this.

> *Anna, a prophetess, was there at the Temple. She was*
> *from the family of Phanuel in the tribe of Asher. She was*
> *now very old. She had lived with her husband seven years*
> *before he died and left her alone. She was now 84 years*
> *old. Anna was always at the Temple; she never left. She*
> *worshiped God by fasting and praying day and night.*
> *Anna was there when Joseph and Mary came to the*
> *Temple. She praised God and talked about Jesus to all*
> *those who were waiting for God to free Jerusalem.*
>
> *Luke 2:36-38*

Our perspective concerning aging and beauty must be aligned with the bible. We have a higher hope in knowing that our earthly bodies are only an outer shell and will one day be replaced with glorified bodies when we take our eternal rest with God in heaven, the real fountain of youth. God is more concerned with our inner beauty than our outer appearance. Let us focus on preparing for our eternal home and dwelling place, rather than focusing on the outer.

> *Do not store up for yourselves treasures on earth, where*
> *moth and rust destroy, and where thieves break in and*
> *steal. But store up for yourselves treasures in heaven,*
> *where neither moth nor rust destroys, and where thieves*

do not break in or steal; where your treasure is, there your heart will be also.

Matthew 6:19-21

Botox is Highly Toxic

The Indian Journal of Dermatology identifies Botulinum toxin, also known as Botox, as one of the most poisonous biological substances known. It is a neurotoxin produced by the bacterium *Clostridium botulinum* [7]. Its use was approved by the FDA in 2002, and classified as a prescription drug to medically treat and cosmetically remove wrinkles [8]. While the name of the drug contains the word toxin, individuals seem oblivious to the fact that what is being injected into their bloodstream is indeed a dangerous toxin.

Because Botox treatments usually only last for 4 to 6 months, individuals must go back to their doctor for more injections. When neurotoxins are injected into the bloodstream, they silently poison and cause damage to the central nervous system and adversely affect functions in both developing and mature nervous tissue. Some of the side effects resulting from Botox treatments are gallbladder dysfunction, respiratory problems, loss of voice, bladder control issues, flu-like symptoms, painful swallowing, drooping eyelids, blurred vision, and fatigue [9]. This is the side of "beauty" that you will not hear about. These treatments are performed out of fear to remove the appearance of getting older. Beauty injections only create the illusion that people are remaining younger and maintaining their beauty when in reality they are not. Botox treatments motivate individuals to be moved solely by what they see, lending themselves over to deception and falsehood, rather than accepting and embracing the true meaning of what it means to age gracefully.

For God has not given us the spirit of fear; but of power, and of love, and of a sound mind.

2 Timothy 1:7

> *For everything in the world—the lust of the flesh, the lust of the eyes, and the pride of life—comes not from the Father but from the world.*
>
> *I John 2:16*

Are Vaccinations Dangerous?

To vaccinate, or not to vaccinate, that is the question. When you strike up a conversation about vaccinations, the topic always generates a heated discussion. From the time we are born, enter Kindergarten, advance on to high school and transition into adulthood, we are required by law to obtain vaccinations; they are considered a normal part of our lives. Growing up as a military brat, and as a retired military veteran, getting vaccinations was a required part of military service. I never questioned the content of the vaccinations being administered and trusted that was being injected into my body was safe. I cannot recall how many vaccinations I have received in all. Just how many vaccinations does an individual receive over the course of their lifetime?

> *As of 2016, the CDC recommends that from birth to age 18, children receive a total of 69 doses of 50 different vaccine injections. Compared to 1983, when children were required to receive a total of 24 doses from a total of 7 vaccine injections.*
>
> *Centers for Disease Control and Prevention*

The above figures do not include vaccinations that are received in adulthood. Although toxic, preservatives have been widely used in biological and drug products, including vaccinations since the 1930's [10]. Multiple doses of preservatives equate to massive amounts of chemicals being released into the bloodstream, overburdening the immune system. The purpose of using preservatives is to prevent potentially life threatening contamination from harmful bacteria or fungi, but it does not guarantee or eliminate the risk of vaccine contamination. One of the most widely used preservatives in vaccines is thimerosal, which is approximately 49.6% mercury by weight. Much like the amalgam fillings mentioned earlier, mercury in any form is toxic and can even be deadly for adults and children when injected into the bloodstream. Because of health concerns associated with thimerosal, manufactures have worked on reducing or eliminating the use of preservatives from vaccines. The FDA vaccine table reveals that several vaccinations to include the influenza shot still contain this preservative [11, 12, 13].

> *The decision to move toward reduced or eliminated thimerosal in vaccines was based on the various Federal guidelines for methyl mercury exposure and the assumption that the health risks from methyl and ethyl mercury were the same.*
>
> *National Institute of Allergy and Infectious Disease*

The effects of methyl mercury poisoning include [14]:

• Central nervous system injury

• Neurological impairment

• Impairment of the peripheral vision

• Adversely effects cognitive thinking, memory, attention, language, and fine motor and visual spatial skills have been seen in children exposed to methyl mercury in the womb

• Disturbances in sensations ("pins and needles" feelings, usually in the hands, feet, and around the mouth)

• Lack of coordination of movements; impairment of speech, hearing, walking; and muscle weakness

In addition to preservatives like thimerosal, vaccinations also contain toxic substances derived from animals and humans. As of 2013, the CDC reported the contents of all vaccines currently being administered to include some of the following:

- Fetal bovine serum (derived from the blood of calf fetus)

- Monkey kidney cells

- Human diploid cells cultures (aborted fetuses or stem cells)

- Madin Darby Canine Kidney (MDCK) cell protein

- Human diploid lung cells

- Embryonic guinea pig cell cultures

- Formaldehyde

- Bovine calf serum

- Chick embryo cell cultures

- Calf serum protein

- Vero cells (DNA from porcine circoviruses or viruses from swine)

The above list is not exhaustive and does not contain nearly half of the contents found in vaccinations [15]. How could anyone honestly believe that any of these substances are deemed safe to inject into any human being? From an ethical standpoint, there is no regard and respect for human and animal life. Under this type of system, individuals are doing what they believe to be right in their own eyes, (Judges 17:6). It is no surprise that the number of new diseases continues to escalate as these substances are injected into our bodies.

> *"I will follow that system of regimen which according to*
> *my ability and judgment I consider best for the benefit*

of my patients and abstain from whatever is deleterious and mischievous."

> **Extract from the Hippocratic Oath,**
> *The World Medical Association Handbook of*
> *Declarations, World Medical Association, Inc.*

It is inconceivable to fathom that this is one of the sinister realities of our current health care system. We have been taught and made to believe that the contents of vaccinations are safe, when in fact they are not. As the Apostle James reminds us, these things should not be so (James 3:10).

> *Our culture believes that it is somehow normal and acceptable to intermingle God's human and animal creations together, along with toxic substances without any negative consequences. To think this way is disconcerting and is a form of inhumane experimentation that is no less than a recipe for disaster.*

The process of manufacturing vaccinations has become unethical and is predominately driven by experimentation, greed, and the love money. The global vaccine industry was valued at 24 billion in 2009 and is estimated to reach 41.85 billion by 2018. Initially, vaccinations were created to guard and protect our health, yet over the years, a dark side of vaccinations has evolved that the public rarely hears about [16, 17].

> *By the close of Fiscal Year 2015, $3,103,832,792.88 (over $3 Billion) in federal compensation has been paid out to children and adults who have been injured or died as a result of vaccinations. Statistics show that 50-75% of applicants that file for federal compensation are denied their claim.*
>
> *National Vaccine Injury Compensation*
> *Program Statistics Report*
>
> *Approximately 30,000 Vaccine Adverse Event Reporting System (VAERS) reports are filed annually, with 10-15%*

classified as serious (resulting in permanent disability, hospitalization, life-threatening illnesses or death).
Centers for Disease Control
and Prevention

Spiritual laws do not change. For whatever a man sows, whether good or bad, in due season a harvest will come forth. Sadly, we are reaping the negative and ill effects of what is being sown through the use of vaccinations. In times like these, we must depend and trust solely on the Lord.

Lean on, trust in, and be confident in the Lord with all your heart and mind and do not rely on your own insight or understanding. In all of your ways know, recognize, and acknowledge Him and he will direct and make straight and plan your paths. Be not wise in your own eyes; reverently fear and worship the lord and turn [entirely] away from evil.
Proverbs 3:5-7

We can no longer remain blindsided about the toxic substances associated with injections that are being transferred into our bloodstreams resulting in impaired health or loss of human life. Living in good health is our God-given birthright and it must be valued and protected.

Build Up Your Immune System

When God created the blood, He created it with what are known as antibodies or antitoxins. Antibodies prevent infection from gaining a foothold in our bodies, while our white blood cells fight off infection as it occurs in the body. Vaccinations contain killed or weakened parts of the germ that is responsible for infection. For example, the flu vaccination contains various strains of the flu virus. When the virus is injected into the bloodstream, the antibodies recognize the infection, increase in large numbers and go to work to kill the virus. However, if the person receiving the vaccination has a weakened immune system, the antibodies and white blood cells are not strong enough to fight off the infection and the individual becomes sick and the vaccination serves no purpose other than contaminating the bloodstream with a virus.

Have you or someone that you know gotten extremely ill after obtaining the flu shot or a vaccination? More than likely, it may have been due to an adverse chemical reaction or a weakened immune system. If an infected person comes in contact with another person with a weakened immune system there is a strong possibility they will become sick. Two of the most vulnerable populations that fall into this category are young children, because their immune systems are still being developed, and the elderly, due to environmental toxins, sedentary lifestyles, and poor eating habits that may have weakened their system. The decline in American health and the increased number of autoimmune disorders and other diseases of the blood puts even more individuals at risk. The CDC makes it clear that there are no guarantees that vaccinations will work based on factors such as age, health, and virus strain matching [18].

> *During years when the flu vaccine is not well matched to circulating viruses, it's possible that no benefit from flu vaccination may be observed. During years when there is a good match between the flu vaccine and circulating viruses, it's possible to measure substantial benefits from vaccination in terms of preventing flu illness. However, even during years when the vaccine match is very good, the benefits of vaccination will vary across the population, depending on characteristics of the person being vaccinated and even, potentially, which vaccine was used.*
> *Centers for Disease Control*
> *and Prevention*

Based on these factors, the process is hit or miss. Vaccinations interfere with the body's natural process of fighting off infection and disease. The most effective and powerful way to build up our immune system is to consistently nourish our blood cells with fresh air, routine exercise, organic whole food, clean water, proper rest, and by cleansing environmental toxins from the blood. By incorporating these lifestyle changes, your body will have the ability to fight off sickness and disease naturally. The promise of health and healing as described in Psalms 91:10 can become a reality in our lives.

No evil shall be allowed to befall you, no plague come near your tent.

Psalms 91:10

A monumental shift is taking place across America concerning vaccinations. Individuals, who value their health, as well as the health of their family, friends, and loved ones, are bravely challenging pharmaceutical companies to re-evaluate the overall safety of vaccines. The National Vaccine Information Center (NVIC) is spearheading such a movement. They have launched a major campaign with the purpose of ensuring vaccine safety and informed consent protection associated with vaccine laws and policies. Informed consent affords individuals the opportunity to voluntarily decline taking a vaccination based on moral or personal beliefs. As believers, spiritual education is essential, but we must also take proactive approaches to becoming informed about important issues that are going on in the world around us.

NVIC is dedicated to the prevention of vaccine injuries and deaths through public education and by defending the informed consent ethic in medicine. This organization does not advocate against the use of vaccines and supports the availability of preventative health care options, including vaccines and the right of consumers to make educated, voluntary health care choices. At the present, the law mandates Americans to obtain vaccinations, even though they may result in sickness, injury, or even death.

Unlike the United Sates, many European countries and other developed countries do not mandate vaccinations for children or adults [19]. As a democratic nation, every individual should be allowed to exercise their liberty to make the decision to choose whether they want vaccinations administered for themselves or loved ones based upon spiritual, physical, moral, or personal reasons. If the contents of vaccinations were proven to be pure, safe, effective, and ethically derived, my stance would be totally different. To knowingly place healthy lives directly in harm's way is immoral and unethical.

The Lord said unto Cain, "Where is your brother Abel? I don't know he replied. Am I my brother's keeper?"

Genesis 4:9

How can men be wise? The only way to begin is by reverence for God. For growth in wisdom comes from obeying his laws. Praise his name forever.

Psalms 111:10

Making Wise Choices to Protect Your Skin

While we are here on this earth, we have one physical body to be good and faithful stewards over. Protecting your skin is vital to your health and is based on making prayerful, educated, and informed decisions. We must be aware of the unknown factors that silently deteriorate our health through the skin. Someday, we will all shed our earthly bodies and cross over into eternity, but while we are here on earth, we can strive to live the quality of life that God has promised us by *Loving, Protecting and Nurturing the Skin* that we're in.

Take care of your body. It's the only place you have to live.

Jim Rohn

Key #2 - Love, Protect & Nurture Your Skin

Healthy Ways to Rock Your Skin Naturally

- If you have obtained tattoos, beauty injections or vaccinations work with a certified holistic health and wellness professional to develop a personal strategy to detoxify your bloodstream to heal and build up your immune system.

- Incorporate alternative beauty treatments to help maintain healthy and youthful skin. Using unrefined organic oils like olive, coconut, almond, and apricot can keep your skin nourished and glowing. These natural oils are saturated with a wealth of essential vitamins and nutrients.

- Integrate massage into your beauty treatment program at least once a month. Massaging the skin promotes deep muscle and tissue relaxation, detoxification, alleviates stress, relieves pain, improves blood circulation, and is beneficial to your overall health and well-being.

- Hydrate your body with plenty of fresh water. Drinking plenty of clean filtered water removes toxins from your body and keeps your skin naturally moisturized and healthy.

- Become educated. Know what's being injected into your bloodstream. Ask your health care provider for a copy of the ingredients in vaccines, as well as any adverse reactions that may be associated. Take time to do some personal research at your local library or medical facility.

- Let your voice be heard on NVIC's Cry for Vaccine Freedom Wall. If you feel that you are receiving ill treatment for choosing not to vaccinate, share your story at www.nvic.org.

- Stay abreast of current vaccine policies and laws by becoming a part of the NVIC team. Invite others who care about their right to make educated decisions about vaccinations by visiting www.nvic.org and click on the Advocacy Portal link to sign up.

* Download the free digital information guide, "Reforming Vaccine Policy and Law" at www.nvic.org This packet will provide you with comprehensive information outlining toxicity dangers, injuries, adverse effects, the truth about this billion-dollar industry and the ineffectiveness of the countless vaccines being administered to children and adults.

Key # 3

*Eat clean organic whole foods and
eliminate processed food.*

[Ingestion / to take in food]

*[Whole food / food which has not been
processed or refined more than is
minimally necessary]*

*So, whether you eat or drink, or whatever you do,
do all to the glory of God.*

1 Corinthians 10:31

Every moving thing that lives shall be meat for you; even as the green herb have I given you all things.
Genesis 9:3

Chapter 5

Is What You're Eating Wrecking Your Healthy World?

What is Food?

God's definition for food is very straightforward, simple and not at all complicated: animals and plant life for food. In the beginning, we were given the responsibility of working in harmony with the earth to cultivate the land to produce crops and raise cattle for food. If you take a quick inventory of what we are eating today, food has taken on many different variations outside of this original definition. Much of what individuals are eating today is not food at all, but a food product.

Food products are highly processed and consist of particles derived from whole foods [1]. Examples of food products are boxed cereal, soda, instant mashed potatoes, donuts, fast food, frozen dinner entrées, jelly, bagels, canned goods, bottled juice, pasta, bread, pastries, ice cream, and potato chips. Basically, any edible item that is not in its original or whole form. This is where the term whole food comes from. Whole food is food that has not been processed, or is minimally processed, and is still in its original whole state. This includes all vegetables, fruits, grains, legumes, and nuts. You might be wondering when did we move away from God's original plan for food? Whole food was transformed into processed food during the Industrial Revolution.

The Industrial Revolution Changed Our Relationship with Food

Not only did the inception of the Industrial Revolution impact our environment, it completely changed our relationship with food. Food that was once commonly grown and harvested by families was suddenly replaced by the mechanical process of canning and packaging food, altering its true form [2]. In order to preserve processed food products, manufactures added salt, sugar, chemicals, fillers, and other additives. The process of canning and packaging food in massive quantities for global distribution became a normal practice and significantly overshadowed the original method of supplying whole food to families.

>*The truth is, processed food is not food in its natural whole form and is nothing more than a food product; this is far from God's original plan regarding food.*

Garbage In, Garbage Out

While serving on Active Duty with the Air Force, one of the jobs that I performed was as a Client System Administrator. I was responsible for troubleshooting computer problems for my organization. One of the first terms that I learned that is still common language in the computer world is GIGO, which stands for Garbage In, Garbage Out. This famous computer axiom means that if invalid information is entered into a computer system, the resulting output will also be invalid [3]. For instance, if a program asked me to enter a certain code that required specific letters from the alphabet and I decide to enter numbers, the result that I would receive back would be "garbage." This would occur because I did not enter or input valid data as required. The human body has been often referenced as the most sophisticated intelligent "computer system" in the world. We must input the right data, in this case whole food, into our bodies to obtain the correct results.

The saying goes, you are what you eat. If you put garbage into your body, the result will ultimately manifest in the form of sickness. Filling our bodies with unhealthy processed food products will always result in GIGO.

The next few sections will focus on the "garbage" found within our food supply, as well as provide strategies on what you can do to keep your body free from it.

Processed Foods and Your Health

When whole food is processed, it is stripped of essential minerals, vitamins, and nutrients, and is converted into a toxic food product with little to no nutritional value. Because our blood cells are living organisms, they need whole living food to stay healthy. Unprocessed, whole foods are considered living food and provide our blood cells with an abundance of nourishment and healing. Processed food products contain no life and are nutritionally dead. Living whole food in the form of fresh fruits and vegetables is natural medicine for the body.

Let food be your medicine and medicine be your food.
Hippocrates

If you've ever taken time to read the ingredients on the back of any popular cereal box or ready-made instant meal, you will discover dozens of nutritionally dead substances, unpronounceable words and questionable ingredients. When substantial amounts of processed foods are consumed, blood cells are contaminated and become damaged, compromising the body's ability to function properly. Eating unhealthy processed food has been correlated to chronic illnesses ranging from obesity, diabetes, asthma, Chronic Fatigue Syndrome, depression, autoimmune disorders, Attention Deficit Hyperactivity Disorder (ADHD), eczema, migraine headaches and insomnia. Because of the health risks associated with eating food products, we must reconsider what we are putting into our bodies.

Pesticides & Your Food

Every person should have access to food that is safe and nourishing. When you visit your local grocery store to shop for produce, you trust that what you are purchasing is just that, safe, and nourishing. Grocery store aisles are lined with brightly colored fresh fruits and vegetables: apples, peppers, carrots, sweet potatoes, and spinach. Outwardly they appear safe, but did you know that almost 100% of the produce being sold to consumers is covered with tasteless and odorless noxious pesticides? Pesticides are poisonous and pose serious health threats to the environment, humans, and animals. The current law allows farmers to use toxic pesticides to help protect crops from pests and diseases. Even when sprayed on plants and food consumed by livestock such as cows, goats, sheep, chickens, or lambs, if humans consume meat from these animals or their byproducts such as butter, eggs, or milk, the pesticides are transferred into the bloodstream. Invisible to the human eye, tests reveal that pesticides are found in more than 90% of Americans bloodstreams due to our contaminated food supply [4,5].

- 93% of Americans tested by the CDC had metabolites of chlorpyrifos neurotoxic insecticide — in their urine. Banned from home use because of its risks to children, chlorpyrifos is part of a family of pesticides (organophosphates) linked to ADHD.

- 99% of Americans tested positive for DDT degradants even though DDT has not been used in the U.S. since 1972. Women who were exposed to DDT as girls are 5 times more likely to develop breast cancer.

Though the federal government regulates the use of pesticides, there are no laws in place prohibiting the use of pesticides. Overwhelming studies show that pesticides have been linked to birth defects, immune disorders, nerve damage, cancer, hormonal imbalances, Parkinson's disease, neurological disorders, and other illnesses that might occur over a long period of time. Pesticides present even greater health risks to children because they are still developing.

In the United States approximately 5.1 billion pounds of pesticides were used in 2006 and 2007. These estimates include conventional pesticides, other chemicals used as pesticides, wood preservatives, specialty biocides, and chlorine/hypochlorites. With more than 2.6 billion pounds used, the amount of chlorine/hypochlorites used was greater than for all other pesticide groups combined.

US Environmental Protection Agency Pesticide Industry Sales and Usage Market Estimates

Since 2007, no new report has been produced by the EPA updating the statistics on the amount of pesticides that are currently being used within our food supply [6]. Strong evidence shows the damaging health effects associated with pesticides and our food, yet they are still being used and almost never is there a link associated with illness and our contaminated food supply.

Alternatives to Pesticide Produce

Many agricultural companies, environmental groups and farmers are committed to not using harmful chemicals and are reverting back to growing food crops, organically. Organic food crops are grown without the use of harmful chemical pesticides, herbicides, and fertilizers. This method relies upon chemical free fertilizers and plant-based herbicides and pesticides and crop rotation to maintain soil productivity and health [7]. Organic crops have proven to be much healthier and safer for human consumption and aid in sustaining our environment. Grocery stores and local farmers markets are providing their communities with a wider selection of organically grown fruits, vegetables, and whole grains. So, how can you tell if what you are purchasing is safe for you and your family?

How to Shop for Organic Produce

Becoming an educated consumer is one of the most important steps that you can take to further guard and protect your divine health. Just as David, you'll have one more stone to slay the giants that are coming against your health. You can determine if produce is organically grown because it will carry the official USDA organic symbol and will also have a label imprinted with a four or five digit code known as the Price Look-up Code or PLU. If the PLU has four digits, and begins with the number 4, it means that it has been conventionally grown, and has been sprayed with pesticides. If the PLU has five digits, beginning with the number 9, it means that the produce was grown organically without the use of pesticides. Here is an example of what the PLU code looks like for a banana:

#4011 - the code for a conventionally grown banana
(harmful chemicals were used)
#94011 - the code for an organically grown banana (harmful chemicals were not used)

One of the main concerns I often hear about is that organic foods cost too much when compared to non-organic foods. Because America is moving towards being a more health-consciousness society, greater availability of organic food is closing the price gap. It's also important to keep in mind that you can never put a price tag on your health. When you are buying organic food, you are paying for high quality, chemical-free food. Buying organically grown food means that you are investing a little more money in your health now, rather than paying for huge medical bills later due to an illness that could have been prevented by simply eating clean food. If you can't afford to buy organic food all of the time, you can strategize by selecting the healthiest and least contaminated food sources for you and your family. Studies have shown that the some of the most contaminated foods that are harmful to human health are: apples, collard greens, bell peppers, blueberries, celery, grapes, kale, peaches, spinach, and strawberries[8]. And with some of the least contaminated foods being: asparagus, avocados, cabbage, cantaloupe, corn, eggplant, mangoes, kiwi, and sweet potatoes[9].

Just as important as ensuring that your food is organically grown, is the need to verify that it is Non-Genetically Modified or Non-GMO.

What Are Genetically Modified Organism (GMO) Foods?

GMOs, have been a part of our food supply for years, yet, most people have no idea they are eating them. The World Health Organization cites that "GMOs are organisms in which genetic material (DNA) has been altered in such a way that does not occur naturally" [10]. For instance, the genes of one species such as a fish are intentionally forced into the natural genetic blueprint of an unrelated plant, like corn or an animal such as a cow, mutating the original gene, thus producing a modified organism. Unfortunately, biotechnology corporations use these modified organisms to manufacture what are known as GMO seeds to grow genetic food crops. Depending on the genetic alteration, the produce that individuals are consuming from these altered seeds may contain genes taken from animals, insects, or bacteria.

God designed every part of creation with a specific purpose. There is a pattern and precise order in the cycle of life. When outside forces begin to deliberately tamper with God's original arrangement and purpose for which an organism was created, disruption is ultimately inevitable. The entire life cycle becomes frustrated and is propelled into a chaotic state.

It was never God's will for anyone to alter His creation. All that God has made is divinely interconnected: man, earth, animals, plant life, and the environment, and when the original blueprint is changed, the connection becomes severely fragmented. Everything in the universe was perfectly aligned and designed and cannot ever be duplicated by man-made means. When God gave the children of Israel laws on agriculture, He specifically told them not to cross-pollinate or modify His originals seeds.

Do not plant your vineyard with two types of seed; otherwise, the entire harvest, both the crop you plant and the produce of the vineyard, will be defiled.

Deuteronomy 22:9

God made it clear that tampering and the intermingling of seeds was prohibited in order to preserve what He had created. Genetically Modified (GM) crops totally go against God's plan and are a warped version of God's original seeds. Although biotechnology corporations may try, they cannot take the place of God, nor can they reproduce what He has created and are operating in what the bible calls foolish wisdom.

For the wisdom of this world is foolishness to God. As the scriptures say, "He traps the wise in the snare of their own cleverness."

1 Corinthians 3:19

Why Are Companies Producing GMO's?

There are many reasons why biotechnology corporations are producing GM crops. To gain a proper perspective, let's take a look at a few of the reasons behind their production [11].

- GM crops have been shown to resist insects, pests, and diseases

- Farmers report experiencing favorable yields from GM crops

- Increased yields results in increased profits for corporations

- Scientists are in control of producing larger crops in a shorter period of time

- GM crops have been shown to last longer and in some cases taste better

GM crops may seem to bring positive benefits, yet there is another side to the seeds that is being unveiled.

GMO's and Our World

As large biotechnology corporations inundate our agricultural landscape with GM crops, the original seeds created by God for food, are rapidly dwindling. GM crops are dominating the food supply, saturating 80% of the American food market [12]. Not only are GM crops being grown in the US, other countries including Argentina, Brazil, China, Canada, India, South Africa, Australia, Paraguay, Uruguay and Europe are also being heavily populated with these altered seeds [13]. As genetic seeds are rapidly funneled into the global market, the short-term and long-term effects on human health and the environment have not been thoroughly investigated. The scriptures remind us that whatever is done secretly will eventually be revealed in the light. This is certainly the case with GM crops as the negative aspects are begin revealed most noticeably within our eco-system.

> *For there is nothing hid, which shall not be manifested; neither was anything kept secret, but that it should be revealed.*
>
> *Mark 4:22*

GMO's and Our Environment

Psalms 104 beautifully describes the eco-system that God created for His people. Man, all living creatures, the environment to include the air, water, and the earth all interact as one large system. We are spiritually linked together and designed to interact harmoniously according to the seasons and cycles on the earth. When one of those links is broken, the eco-system becomes greatly impaired. Season after season, our eco-system is kept in balance as vegetable and fruit crops are pollinated by insects and creatures such as butterflies, moths, flies, beetles, birds, bats, and honey bees. Pollination of all plant life is necessary to replenish the earth with new seeds and to supply it with fresh vegetation to continue and complete the life cycle. Because GM crops are engineered to resist insects and pests, they stop the natural process of pollination from occurring. The ramifications of stopping pollination have rippling effects more far reaching than we could ever fathom.

> *The land produced vegetation, all sorts of seed-bearing plants, and trees with seed-bearing fruit. Their seeds produced plants and trees of the same kind. And God saw that it was good.*
>
> *Genesis 1:12*

New seeds are crucial to producing the next generation of plant life to sustain life on earth. Grassroots organizations, local farmers, health educators and politicians are breaking the silence about the damaging ecological impact of GM seeds. The award-winning documentary, "Vanishing of the Bees" provides invaluable insight concerning the phenomenon known as Colony Collapse Disorder, the rapid loss of the adult honeybee population within our eco-system [14]. The massive death of honey bees reveals that our current food system has become highly unsustainable through engineering methods and industrial practices that are being used to grow food. Pollination is crucial to our continued existence due to the fact that honey bees pollinate 1 out of every 3 bites of whole food. Without pollination, to produce new plant life, the cycle of life is being propelled into a devastatingly chaotic state, impacting our supply of oxygen, food, clothing, shelter, and medicine.

Furthermore, GM crops are producing what are known as "super weeds" and "super bugs" which can only be killed with toxic herbicides engineered by biotechnology companies such as Roundup [15]. Charles Benbrook, a research professor at the Center for Sustaining Agriculture and Natural Resources at Washington State University, disclosed that from 1996 to 2001, the use of pesticides insecticides, fungicides, herbicides, rodenticides, and weedicides, have led to a 404 million pound increase in overall pesticide use since the introduction of GM crops, further contaminating our food supply and polluting the earth's natural resources [16]. Not only are GMO's harmful to environmental health, they are also damaging to human health.

GMO's and Your Health

Our bloodstream is considered to be an environment that is well separated from the outside world. Based on a study conducted at Yale School of Public Health, over 1,000 human samples from four independent studies show that when GM foods are consumed they are easily assimilated into our bloodstream[17]. Intermingling genetically modified substances with human DNA produces confusion within the body and results in a number of health issues. Through the organization Environmental Sciences Europe, scientists examined the health impacts of rats eating commercialized genetically modified maize, alongside of the herbicide Roundup and found severe liver and kidney damage, hormonal disturbances, a high rate of large tumors and mortality in most treatment groups. Further validating the damaging health effects of GM food, the Institute of Responsible Technology conducted an investigative study linking five health conditions that include autoimmune disorders, gluten-related disorders and Celiac Disease affecting over 18 million Americans[18, 19].

- Damage to intestinal wall

- Impaired digestion

- Immune activation and allergic response

- Imbalanced gut and

- Intestinal permeability

Due to the negative effects of GMO's food, twenty-six countries have banned them from their country to include Russia[20, 21].

> *"It is necessary to ban GMOs, to impose a moratorium (on) it for 10 years. While GMOs will be prohibited, we can plan experiments, tests, or maybe even new methods of research could be developed. It has been proven that not only in Russia, but also in many other countries in the world, GMOs are dangerous. Methods of obtaining the GMOs are not perfect, therefore, at this stage, all GMOs are dangerous. Consumption and use of GMOs obtained in such way can lead to tumors, cancers, and obesity among*

animals. Biotechnologies certainly should be developed, but GMOs should be stopped. We should stop it from spreading."

Irina Ermakova, VP of Russia's
National Association for Genetic Safety

Biotechnology company's efforts to produce healthier food in shorter periods of time have resulted in successfully engineering what is no less than a Weapon of Mass Destruction, proliferating biologically, chemically, genetically, and environmentally on unimaginable levels. From the beginning time, God has always had a set order for all of creation that cannot be changed, not even by man. King Solomon summed it up best when he penned the following words of wisdom:

To everything there is a season, and a time for every matter or purpose under heaven:
A time to be born and a time to die, a time to plant and a time to pluck up what is planted,
A time to kill and a time to heal, a time to break down and a time to build up,
A time to weep and a time to laugh, a time to mourn and a time to dance,
A time to cast away stones and a time to gather stones together, a time to embrace and a time to refrain from embracing,
A time to get and a time to lose, a time to keep and a time to cast away,
A time to rend and a time to sew, a time to keep silence and a time to speak,
A time to love and a time to hate, a time for war and a time for peace.

Ecclesiastes 3:1-10

Spiritually and naturally, operating within the original designs, patterns, and cycles is the only way that we can survive on the earth. Scientific research has continually proven that GM crops have never, nor do they show any signs of yielding positive results, making this type of process to grow food unethical and unsustainable. Becoming knowledgeable about what you are eating is imperative to your health. Essentially, your life and the life of future generations depend on it. While biotechnology corporations are becoming wealthier, and health care costs continue to soar, know that all is not lost. There is a way of escape. You can take immediate action on a personal level by refusing to support this system by turning back to God's plan for health. Our times may have changed, but God's ways have never changed.

I am the Lord thy God and I do not change.
Malachi 3:6a

The safest and healthiest practice for you, your family and the environment is to purchase food that is prominently marked with the following information:

1) The USDA Organic symbol

2) Non-GMO verified symbol

3) A PLU number beginning with the number nine for organic verification

Ensure that the food you are purchasing is from trusted sources. Trusted sources include locally grown food from farmers, health food stores and growing your own food with organic non-GMO seeds or heirloom seeds. Heirloom seeds are seeds that have been passed down for generations in a particular region or area. These seeds are open-pollinated, which means they are pollinated by insects, creatures, or wind without human intervention. Now that you have a clear understanding about why eating the right kind of produce matters, we'll also take a look at why eating the right kind of meat is just as important.

Why Eating Humanely Raised Meat Matters

Overcrowded cages, inhumane slaughtering practices, disease infested conditions, antibiotic, and hormone injections administered by the thousands, exposure to high levels of greenhouse emissions, unhealthy GM diets, gross maltreatment, unsanitary practices and rodent infested living environments. These are dreadful circumstances that no creature should ever have to experience. These are the horrific surroundings that animals are subjected to living in for the course of their entire lives before reaching super markets and finally into our homes. It is understandable why so many individuals are choosing to become vegetarians. Much like the produce industry, the meat industry has become desperately wicked and has been taken over by invisible forces of darkness ruled by corporate greed. Billions of dollars are generated annually, as God's creatures are appallingly devalued and callously mistreated. In response to this inhumane treatment, undercover investigators across the nation are taking bold and courageous action by capturing video footage of the most unimaginable atrocities that animals must endure.

> *For our wrestling is not against flesh and blood, but against the principalities, against the powers, against the world-rulers of this darkness, against the spiritual hosts of wickedness in the heavenly places.*
>
> *Ephesians 6:12*

Even if animals are sickly or disease ridden with tumors, they are seen as nothing more than a commodity and their meat is still sold to the market for human consumption. Meat is soaked and injected with a number of toxic chemicals to sanitize it or it is dyed with pigmentation to make its appearance more appealing prior to packaging. If you are not eating meat that is humanely raised, not only are you consuming the myriad of toxins absorbed by the animal, you are also ingesting the trauma, sickness, and torture that these animals had to endure. Just as fruits, vegetables, and grains are being labeled with organic and Non-GMO seals, the same practice is being implemented for meat through the Animal Welfare Rating Standards system. Global Animal Partnership is a non-profit organization that is dedicated to preserving the well-being of farm raised animals [22]. They have developed a 5-Step Animal Welfare Rating Standard that rates how chickens and their eggs, cattle, pigs, and turkeys are raised for human consumption.

When purchasing meat, be sure to look for this rating system to know how the animals were raised. Each rating is clearly marked with a bright orange, yellow, or green square label ranging from steps one through five. Some farm and ranch owners even provide links to their web site on the packaging to give you a virtual tour of their farm. Here's how the rating system works [23].

> **Step 1** - No crates, no cages and no crowding. Animals live with adequate space to freely move around and stretch their legs.
> **Step 2** - Enriched environment. Animals are provided with lifestyle enhancements to help them engage in their natural behavior. For example, chickens are provided with bales of straw to peck at.
> **Step 3** - Enhanced outdoor access. Animals may live in buildings, but they are all afforded the opportunity to have access to outdoor areas to get some fresh air.
> **Step 4** - Pasture centered. Animals live in enriched outdoor environments giving them plenty of fresh air and space. Animals regularly rotate pastures to ensure they are getting the most nutrient rich grasses and to allow the land to recover between grazing.
> **Step 5** - Animal centered approach. This step ensures that priority is placed on the welfare of the animal. Any physical alterations such as branding are prohibited.
> **Step 5+** - The entire life of the animal is spent on one farm.

Through Global Animal Partnership, the 5-Step program includes 2,800+ farms and ranches, and 290 million animals have been certified as humanely raised. Knowing that you are purchasing and eating meat that has been raised humanely is extremely important for animal, human and environmental health. The 5-Step system provides an exceptional stepping-stone that enables our country to work together for a healthier

America. To enhance this system even further, labeling to include non-genetic engineering of meat must also be considered.

Genetically Engineered Meat and Fish

In 2010, a national survey conducted by Lake Research, revealed that Americans strongly believe that the FDA should not approve genetically engineered meat or fish for human consumption until more research is completed [24].

- 78% of Americans oppose genetically engineered meat and/or fish

- 16% of Americans want to see it approved

- 6% of Americans are unsure

Currently no genetically engineered fish or meat products have been approved for food production in the United States. To date only one company, has publicly announced that it has requested FDA approval to market a genetically engineered food animal, a growth-enhanced Atlantic salmon, capable of growing 4 to 6 times faster than standard salmon grown under the same conditions. If the FDA approves the request to genetically engineer fish, it will no doubt open the doorway for even more animal engineering to include cattle, turkey, chickens, pigs, goats, and lambs etc. Based on the poor performance of GM food crops, this same harmful trend could develop from animal engineering. One of the ways to respond to this is by collectively changing the laws to mandate proper Genetic Engineering (GE) labeling.

It's Time to Change the Law

At the present, there are no Federal laws mandating the use labels to show that food contains GE ingredients. Non-GMO labeling currently takes place at the state level. Implementing labeling on the Federal level would create a more universal and streamlined process for our country.

In April 2014, bill S.809, also known as the Genetically Engineered Food Right-to-Know-Act was introduced to the Senate by Senator Barbra Boxer [D-CA] [25]. The bill requests that current FDA regulations be amended to properly label any food for human consumption that has been genetically engineered or contains one or more genetic ingredients unless such information is clearly disclosed. Although no movement has taken place on the bill, the voices of the American people must be heard. To view bill S.809 in its entirety, you can do so by visiting http://www.congress.gov. In the search box at the top of the page type bill number S.809. You can electronically send your comments to your local Congressional leader and Senator to share your thoughts about why changing this bill into a law is necessary for preserving the health of our nation. As consumers, we have a legal right to know what we are eating. While it can take quite some time for laws to change, let us remain prayerful, hopeful, and actively engaged, trusting that the laws will change in favor of our health.

Eating Is a Spiritual Practice

Christians have disconnected the way that we eat from our spirituality, when in fact God ordained eating as a spiritual practice. When God originally prescribed laws to the children of Israel in the book of Leviticus concerning eating, He made it known that there is a distinction concerning what food He wanted us to eat; organic whole foods and clean meats. In addition to what we are to eat, God also shared that we are not to overindulge in gluttonous eating habits.

> *"...and put a knife to your throat if you are given to appetite."*
>
> *Proverbs 23:2*

Our nation has become one that is obsessed with doing everything in an enormous or extravagant way. Bigger cars, larger houses and when it comes to eating, we are given the option to biggie size or super size every meal. The convenience of overindulging in unhealthy, oversized fast food meal portions has contributed to America's 52% obesity rate. The fat, sugar, and chemical content in these food products inflict damage to our blood cells, creating a chain reaction, plaguing the body with diseases such as high blood pressure, inflammation, stroke, arthritis, heart disease and cancer. Most restaurants use a variety of unhealthy cooking methods that change the chemical composition of food, which include: microwaving, frying, barbequing, pan searing, and grilling. When eaten, they further harm and change the chemical composition of your blood cells. The ease of purchasing fast food products and eating out at restaurants 4-5 times out of the week has literally replaced preparing, healthier home cooked meals [26].

> *"In 1970, Americans spent about $6 billion on fast food; in 2000, they spent more than $110 billion. Americans now spend more money on fast food than on higher education, personal computers, computer software, or new cars. They spend more on fast food than on movies, books, magazines, newspapers, videos, and recorded music combined."*
>
> *Fast Food Nation, The Dark Side of the All-American Meal Eric Schlosser*

With fewer meals being prepared at home, there is no control over proper food preparation or sanitary practices. Not disinfecting food equipment and utensils, improper hand washing, poor hygiene and improper food preparation have all been traced back to food borne illnesses. The CDC estimates that each year roughly 1 in 6 Americans or 48 million people get sick, 128,000 are hospitalized, and 3,000 die from foodborne diseases [27].

It's Time to Think About What You Are Eating

We put ourselves at a great disadvantage when we wastefully spend our financial resources on food products that contribute to sickness, yet day in and day out, our culture consumes staggering amounts of unhealthy toxic food. We are simply not taking the time to think about what we are eating on a spiritual level. Rather than embracing a whole food lifestyle as prescribed in the bible, we are consuming dangerous food substances that were never meant to be eaten.

Daniel, Hananiah, Mishael and Azariah are prime examples of making decisions based upon biblical principles concerning our eating. Because their choices stemmed from their obedience and love for God, they experienced amazing health and were found to be unparalleled in wisdom, spiritual agility, interpretation of dreams, leadership ability and were also gifted in mathematics and the sciences. Further proving that eating biblically has everything to do with how we function mentally, emotionally, spiritually, and physically.

> *Daniel spoke with the attendant who had been appointed by the chief of staff to look after Daniel, Hananiah, Mishael, and Azariah. Please test us for ten days on a diet of vegetables and water, Daniel said. "At the end of the ten days, see how we look compared to the other young men who are eating the king's food. Then make your decision in light of what you see. The attendant agreed to Daniel's suggestion and tested them for ten days. At the end of the ten days, Daniel and his three friends looked healthier and better nourished than the young men who had been eating the food assigned by the king. So after that, the attendant fed them only vegetables instead of the food and wine provided for the others.*
>
> *Daniel 1:11-15*

The various methods in which we prepare and grow food may have changed, but God's plan for food has never changed. His plan has always been simplistic in nature, yet is deeply embedded with spiritual principles. When followed, God's way leads to living a healthy life overflowing with vitality and strength.

The recurring cycle of mindless eating in America is totally dependent upon our five physical senses, what we can see, smell, hear, touch, and taste, rather than on the biblically centered spiritual side of eating. This physical sensed type of eating leads us to believe that if it looks, tastes, and smells good, then it must be good for me. This is a fallacy. The bible reminds us that we have the mind of Christ, therefore, as His children, we have taken on His nature and can think and operate the way that Jesus did on the earth, even in relation to our eating. In our thinking, we must begin developing a disciplined mindset to make wise choices that are pleasing to God that will in turn benefit our health.

> *I call heaven and earth to witness this day against you that I have set before you life and death, the blessings and the curses; therefore choose life, that you and your descendants may live.*
>
> *Deuteronomy 30:19*

When and if you go out to eat, begin asking yourself some of these basic questions to redirect your relationship with food: Is what I'm eating being driven solely by my physical senses? Am I eating whole food or a food product? Am I eating the healthiest food choice for my body? Where did the food come from? What methods were used to prepare the food i.e. microwave, fried, barbequed, grilled? How was it processed? Was it humanely raised? Is it Genetically Modified? These questions will help you to begin thinking mindfully about what you are eating. Your very health rests on these questions. Not only do we need to deeply consider what we are eating, we must take into account how we are eating.

How We Are Eating Is Important

All too often, food is eaten hurriedly usually while driving, watching television, working on the computer, walking down the street or multi-tasking. Whenever the bible speaks of eating food, it speaks of people sitting down and breaking bread together. During an evening meal, while Jesus was sitting down at a table relaxing with His disciples, Matthew 26:20-30, says that He took bread, praised God, gave thanks, broke it, blessed it and gave it to his disciples. In the book of Revelations, God describes a beautiful picture of the marriage supper that Christians will enjoy with Him in our new heavenly home.

> *Let us rejoice and be glad and give the glory to Him, for the marriage of the Lamb has come and His bride has made herself ready. It was given to her to clothe herself in fine linen, bright and clean; for the fine linen is the righteous acts of the saints. Then he said to me,*

> *"Write, blessed are those who are invited to the marriage*
> *supper of the Lamb." And he said to me, "These are true*
> *words of God."*
>
> *Revelation 19:7-9*

Christians will be seated at a royal banquet table that could only be fashioned by the Father Himself. How we are eating truly is important to God. He never intended for us to wolf down food and drink. Just as Jesus gave thanks for the food that was before Him, God wants us to follow this example by enjoying and appreciating the true blessing and gift of food. It is time for the Body of Christ to return to God's principles concerning our eating. He has graciously blessed us by abundantly filling the earth with organic whole foods and humanely raised meats that are healing, nutritious, and delicious. God takes great delight and is honored when we partake of the blessings that He has provided to us.

> *Day by day continuing with one mind in the temple, and*
> *breaking bread from house to house, they were taking*
> *their meals together with gladness and sincerity of heart,*
> *praising God and having favor with all the people. And*
> *the Lord was adding to their number day by day those*
> *who were being saved.*
>
> *Acts 2:46-47*

Eating and Your Blood Type Diet

Did you know that one of the fundamentals of disease-free living could be as simple as understanding and knowing your blood type? During my studies as a health coach, diet and nutrition were the foundation of my curriculum. I studied over 100 dietary theories and concepts about different foods and diets, and their impact on an individual's overall health and wellness. I began to understand that bio-individuality is something that is all too often overlooked when addressing wellness needs. When I began working with clients, why did one method of dieting work for one person and fail for another? Initially, I did not realize that it had to do with our different blood types, further validating what God shared with me in Leviticus 17:11. Just as each person possesses unique qualities specific to his or her DNA, so it is with our health. Our biological differences, determine what we need to experience vibrant health.

> *One man's food is another man's poison.*
> *Titus Lucretius Carus*

I discovered that creating wellness plans specific to my client's needs based on their blood type consistently produced positive results. The Blood Type Diet, created by Dr. Peter J. D'Adamo, focuses on eating nourishing whole foods and quality proteins that react chemically with your blood type in one of the four categories: O, A, AB and A [28]. When followed, food is digested more efficiently, energy levels are increased and blood cells are nourished with specific foods for disease prevention.

> **Type O blood:** A high protein diet that focuses on lean meat, poultry, fish, and vegetables, and light on grains, beans, and dairy.

> **Type A blood:** A meat-free diet based on fruits and vegetables, legumes, and whole grains—ideally, organic, and fresh.

> **Type B blood:** Focuses on eating green vegetables, eggs, certain meats, and low-fat dairy are highly beneficial.

> **Type AB blood:** Foods to focus on include tofu, seafood, dairy, and green vegetables.

If you don't know what your blood type is, you may be able to obtain it by contacting your primary care doctor or you can donate blood at your local American Red Cross.

God's Way is Always the Best Way

As we look around our world today, there is no doubt that we are living in the end times. God needs His people well spiritually and physically for the days that lie ahead. We must be fit to fight for the

Kingdom of God. We have come to a point in time where we must lay down our own wisdom and reconnect our spirituality back to God's way of eating, because what we are doing in our own strength is simply not working. When God gave us the key of eating clean, GMO free, organic whole foods in Genesis 3:19, somehow, over the course of time we discarded it, choosing another way. The wonderful thing about God is that He understands and recognizes that in our humanity we will make mistakes. It is His amazing grace that offers us the opportunity to pick up the keys again so that we can live a life overflowing with health. When we follow His path, we have the promise of living and experiencing a life that is most blessed.

> *[Most] blessed is the man who believes in, trusts in, and relies on the Lord, and whose hope and confidence the Lord is. For he shall be like a tree planted by the waters that spreads out its roots by the river; and it shall not see and fear when heat comes; but its leaf shall be green. It shall not be anxious and full of care in the year of drought, nor shall it cease yielding fruit.*
>
> *Jeremiah 17:7-8*

Key # 3 - Eat Clean Non-GMO Organic Whole Food and Eliminate Processed Food

Healthy Ways to Rock Your World Naturally with Clean Eating

- Commit to eating according to God's plan by purchasing and including more organic, Non-GMO whole foods into your daily meals.

- Become an educated consumer by reading food labels to know what you are eating. If you cannot pronounce an ingredient, more than likely, it is not healthy for consumption.

- Before eating ensure that you say a prayer and give thanks to God for the blessing and gift of food.

- To find out how you can support local farmers and ranches and the protection of farm-raised animals visit Global Animal Partnership's web site http://www. globalanimalpartnership.org.

- If you choose to consume meat, ensure that it is humanely raised. If your grocery store does not use the 5-Step Animal Welfare Rating System, ask the store manager how this can be implemented.

- Develop a plan to prepare and cook meals at home versus eating out at restaurants or fast-food chains. To make the experience more enjoyable and memorable invite family, friends, or neighbors to join you.

- Join the Non-GMO Project movement by visiting http://www. nongmoproject.org. Once on the site, you can find out how you can shop Non-GMO, make a product verification request, find retailers that support the Non-GMO Project movement or donate to help support the Non-GMO Project.

- Learn more about honey bees and their critical role in sustaining our food supply by visiting www.vanishingofthebees.com.

- Download the Environmental Working Group's Healthy Living app. This app will help you to select healthy, clean whole food options for you and your family.

- Opt to cook at home. If you're new to cooking, sign up to take a free healthy cooking class at your local library, church, or community center.

- Avoid the temptation of buying fast food by packing healthy breakfast food i.e. herbal tea, oatmeal, sandwich wraps, fresh fruit or nut trail mix when on the go or to take to work. This will also help you to save money. Track your savings to see how much money you are saving every week.

Key # 4

*Drink clean filtered water to keep
the body hydrated and operating at optimal levels.*

[Ingestion / to take in water]

*[Water / the colorless, transparent,
odorless, tasteless liquid that forms the seas, lakes, rivers,
and rain and is the basis of the fluids of all
living organisms]*

*You visit the earth and saturate it with water; You
greatly enrich it; the river of God is full of water;
You provide them with grain when
You have so prepared the earth.*

Psalms 65:9

*You water the field's furrows abundantly, You settle the ridges of it;
You make the soil soft with showers, blessing the sprouting of
its vegetation. You crown the year with Your bounty and goodness,
and the tracks of Your [chariot wheels] drip with fatness. The
[luxuriant] pastures in the uncultivated country drip [with moisture],
and the hills gird themselves with joy. The meadows are clothed
with flocks, the valleys also are covered with grain;
they shout for joy and sing together.*
Psalms 69:10-13

Chapter 6

Water: The Essential Nutrient for Life

W ater. It's all around us. It's one of the first elements recorded in the bible.

*When the earth was as yet unformed and desolate, with
the surface of the ocean depths shrouded in darkness, and
while the Spirit of God was hovering over the surface of
the waters.*

Genesis 1:2

Water covered the face of the earth even before we existed; a perfectly crafted combination of hydrogen and oxygen, producing one of our most

119

invaluable resources. Water covers over 70% of the earth's surface and is used in our everyday lives for drinking, agriculture, recreation, washing, energy production, cooking, and cleaning [1]. Our oceans, seas, lakes, streams, rivers, waterfalls, clouds, and atmosphere are all comprised of this tasteless and odorless substance. Water is the only element that can be readily transformed into three separate states: liquid, solid, and gas.

In liquid form, water serves as oxygen and provides habitation for billions of aquatic animals and plant life. In extremely cold regions, like the Arctic, frozen water serves as home for a diverse population of animal species such as polar bears, Arctic foxes, whales, penguins, seals, and snow geese. When clouds accumulate enough water in a gaseous state, it is released back onto the earth in the form of raindrops. All of creation could not survive without the existence of water.

> *And God said, Let there be an expanse in the midst of the waters, and let it separate the waters from the waters. And God made the expanse and separated the waters that were under the expanse from the waters that were above the expanse. And it was so.*
>
> *Genesis 1:6-8*
>
> *By his knowledge the depths are broken up, and the clouds drop down the dew.*
>
> *Proverbs 3:20*

Water is a Vital Nutrient

Water is an extremely vital nutrient, and is more than just a liquid substance to satisfy thirst. No other fluid matter outside of water can supply the body with an abundance of nutrition, energy, life, and strength to support its overall survival and development. The brain and heart are composed of 73% water, and the lungs are about 83% water. The skin contains 64% water, muscles, and kidneys are 79%, and even the bones are 31% water [2]. Because our bodies primarily consist of water, a multitude of operations cannot function properly without it [3]. Water is responsible for:

- Helping the heart to easily pump blood through vessels

- Regulating body temperature

- Lubricating and cushioning joints

- Protecting body tissue and organs

- Carrying nutrients and oxygen to cells

- Moistening tissues such as those in the mouth, eyes, and nose

- Helping to prevent constipation

- Preventing premature aging by keeping the cells healthy

- Aids in naturally detoxing and cleansing the body

- Improving memory, focus, and concentration

- Metabolizing nutrients and minerals

- Improving overall tissue function

- Flushing out the kidneys and bladder

- Removing toxins from the body

All systems in the body to include brain function, nervous system, vital organs and the bloodstream are dependent upon water. When God created water, He knew that it would be the healthiest liquid to sustain human health. Drinking water aids the bloodstream to flow freely and flushes out toxins within the blood. Without drinking water, the buildup of toxins in the bloodstream cannot be removed and creates an unhealthy and highly toxic environment for infections, bacteria, fungus, and parasites to thrive. The ultimate purpose of drinking water is to keep the body cleansed, balanced, and healthy.

Americans Are Simply Not Drinking Enough Water

A study conducted by the Centers for Disease Control and Prevention reveals that 43% of adults drink less than four cups of water a day. That includes 36% who drink one to three cups, and 7 % who drink no water at all [4,5,6]. Because individuals are not supplying the body with the nutrients that it needs by drinking water, various illnesses manifest in many forms:

- Cancer

- Depression

- Sleeping issues

- Headaches

- Brain fog

- Low energy

- Brain fatigue

- Asthma

- Dry mouth

- Chronic aches and pains

- High blood pressure

- Poor digestion

- Chronic fatigue

- Poor memory and concentration

- Irregular blood sugar levels (leading to diabetes)

• Eating disorders (Anorexia, bulimia, and binge eating)

Water was created as a natural healing agent and when the body is fully nourished with it, many illnesses are highly preventable and reversible. Instead of prescribing medications, one simple solution to aid in naturally healing the body would be to simply drink water.

> *Unfortunately, the first line of defense when treating physical symptoms is to prescribe medication. The manifestation of symptoms may not be illness at all, but may serve as an indicator that they body is actually thirsty for water.*

If water is so vital to our health, why aren't people drinking more of it? The main reason rests upon the taste; water has no flavor.

Choosing Flavor Over Health

Stacks of aluminum, glass, and plastic bottles filled with soda, energy drinks, coffee, tea, and juice saturate supermarkets, movie theaters, vending machines, restaurants, and convenient stores. These drinks contain some form of water, but are also full of toxic chemicals, dyes, preservatives, and artificial sweeteners. Of these ingredients, the sweet taste of sugar is the driving force that compels individuals to keep going back for more of their favorite flavored drink.

Research conducted by the American Heart Association shows that the average American consumes more than 100 pounds of sugar and sweeteners per year. Most of this sugar is consumed in what we are drinking [7]. The recommended amount of sugar consumption in any form, natural or artificial sweetener, per day for women is no more than 6 teaspoons or 100 calories and no more than 9 teaspoons or 150 calories for men. Most Americans are eating and drinking about 22 teaspoons per day—that's significantly more than the recommended daily value [8].

The Problem with Consuming Too Much Sugar

Refined sugar provides no nutritional value to the body and suppresses the immune system. Studies show that sugar is highly addictive and is no different than anyone facing a cocaine, heroin, or alcohol addiction [9]. One of the most common problems that I witness among clients involves consuming a combination of food and drinks that equate to large amounts of sugar being released into the bloodstream. For instance, if a person consumes orange juice, frosted cereal, a bagel with jelly, coffee with sugar, two candy bars, ice-cream, pastries, and a few sodas over the course of one day, they have more than exceeded the recommended daily amount of sugar. If someone drinks one can of soda, they've just consumed 35 grams of sugar, equivalent to 8.75 teaspoons of sugar. One of the main factors contributing to the declining health of Americans is the overconsumption of sugar. Individuals believe that when their energy levels are low, eating, or drinking something sweet will make them feel better, and boost their energy level, giving them the extra charge they need to make it through the day. Truthfully, sugar does provide a temporary boost of energy, but once the body comes off of the "sugar high," blood sugar levels drops and the body is conditioned to crave more sugar, causing a sugar addiction. Knowing and giving your body what it needs is paramount to breaking the cycle of consuming sugar-sweetened drinks and food. To experience health at a greater level, sugar consumption must decrease and the habit of drinking water must increase.

It's Time to Upgrade Your Fuel

Just as high octane grade fuel is to a luxury automobile, so water is to the body. Putting a lower grade fuel into a luxury car can prove to be harmful to the engine. Your body is no different. You are fearfully and wonderfully made. Continually filling your body with a lower grade of fuel, sugar-sweetened and caffeinated drinks will end up ruining your health. Consuming too many sugary drinks is a serious factor, contributing to the health crisis in America.

The Effects of Sugar on Your Blood Cells

Too much sugar in the bloodstream coats your red blood cells, causing them to become stiff. The stickiness of the cells interferes with blood circulation and causes cholesterol to build up on the inside of your blood vessels. It can take months or even years for the damage to appear in your body. Delicate blood vessels located in your eyes, feet, kidneys, and eyes become impaired and are affected the most. The effects of sugar weakens blood cells, breaking down the immune system, leaving it with no strength to ward off sickness and disease. Because the blood is comprised of living cells, it cannot assimilate artificial sweeteners, chemicals, and toxins, much of what sugary drinks are composed of. To further validate the ills associated with sugar, below are 20 key reasons adapted from the book, *146 Reasons Why Sugar is Ruining Your Health,* by Nancy Appleton, PhD [10].

1. Sugar can suppress the immune system.

2. Sugar interferes with absorption of calcium and magnesium.

3. Sugar can weaken eyesight.

4. Sugar can cause hypoglycemia.

5. Sugar can cause a rapid rise of adrenaline levels in children.

6. Sugar contributes to obesity.

7. Sugar can cause arthritis.

8. Sugar can cause heart disease and emphysema.

9. Sugar can contribute to osteoporosis.

10. Sugar can increase cholesterol.

11. Sugar can lead to both prostate cancer and ovarian cancer.

12. Sugar can contribute to diabetes.

13. Sugar can cause cardiovascular disease.

14. Sugar can make our skin age by changing the structure of collagen.

15. Sugar can produce a significant rise in triglycerides.

16. Sugar can increase the body's fluid retention.

17. Sugar can cause headaches, including migraines.

18. Sugar can cause depression.

19. Sugar can contribute to Alzheimer's disease.

20. In intensive care units, limiting sugar saves lives.

Do Not Despise the Blessing of Water

Unlike other countries, America is truly blessed to have access to clean drinking water. We can walk into our kitchen or bathroom and turn on the faucet and the water flows within a few seconds. Throughout my military travels, I have lived in countries where homes had no running water. It was normal to see people carrying buckets to local community pumps to obtain water for drinking, cooking, and bathing. These experiences taught me about being grateful and appreciative for every blessing that God has given to us [11].

> *About 2.6 billion people – half the developing world have no access to any type of improved drinking source of water. Of these, 1.6 million people die every year from diseases attributable to lack of access to safe drinking*

*water and basic sanitation and 90% of these are children
under five, mostly in developing countries.*
World Health Organization

In America, we have been blessed with so much, and at times, I sense that we have turned the blessing into a curse. Meaning that, because we have been given so much, we take for granted what we have been blessed with. We are surrounded with the abundant blessing of water. Growing up, I often heard my mother echo the familiar adage, "You never miss your water until the well runs dry." Imagine what our entire country would be like if we woke up one day and were without water. Our nation would come to a screeching halt. We must begin to reframe our thinking, as well as retrain our taste buds to begin enjoying the true blessing and gift of water.

How Much Water Do You Need to Drink?

When it comes down to the amount of water that you should drink, there is not a formula that fits everyone. We all live different lifestyles with some being more active than others. Drinking too little water can create health problems and drinking too much can create a mineral imbalance within the body. Your daily water intake is based upon a number of various factors such as your activity, height, weight, body chemistry, eating habits, the climate you live in and how healthy you are.

Knowing how much water you need is determined by learning how to listen to your body. When you feel the urge to reach for a soda or energy drink, this is your body signaling that it is lacking nutrients that can only be satisfied by drinking water. If you need a figure to gauge your daily water intake, The Institute of Medicine, on average, recommends that men should ingest about 3 liters (13 cups) and women about 2.2 liters (9 cups) of water each day [12]. Water can also be absorbed into the body by eating fresh fruit, green leafy vegetables and homemade broths and by juicing and/or blending fruits and vegetables. If you are consistently drinking or eating organic whole fruits and vegetables, most likely you will not need as much water as someone who has poor eating habits consisting largely of processed foods. Sodas and other sugar-sweetened drinks do not count towards your daily water intake because they do not contain the healing properties found in plain water. If you want to begin drinking more water, and want to get past the taste of plain water, there are a variety of ways to add flavor.

- Add fresh mint leaves

- Add a squeeze or slice of lemon or lime

- Sliced cucumbers add a refreshing zing

- Enjoy water as a warm herbal tea (passion fruit, dandelion, ginger)

- Make a healing vegetable broth (carrots, broccoli, onions, parsley)

- Freeze fresh fruit and use it as ice cubes (oranges, blueberries, raspberries, or cherries)

- Infuse water with fresh fruit (pineapple chunks, strawberries, blueberries, kiwi, or limes)

- Add a splash of 100% fruit juice (cranberry, apple, or pomegranate)

Again, the key to knowing whether or not you are getting enough water is learning how to listen to your body. Some of the most common signals that your body is dehydrated are: dark and fowl smelling urine, dry mouth, very dry skin, hunger pains even though you have already eaten, constipation, fatigue, and back pain [13]. Try this experiment. If you are still feeling hungry after a meal, instead of eating more food or drinking a soda, drink a glass of water. If you're still feeling hungry or thirsty, you may need to seek out additional nutritional support to help you pinpoint where your thirst or cravings are coming from.

> *Your body has a language. When it speaks give it what it needs and not what you want. Clean water, proper rest,*

fresh air, exercise, and nourishing whole food. These basic habits are the cornerstone to living a healthy lifestyle.

Hot, Cold, or Room Temperature...What Is the Best Way to Drink Water?

Millions of people start their day gulping down extremely hot or icy cold beverages. If you pick up coffee or tea before going to work at any fast food establishment or convenient store, all hot cups are pre- printed with large warning labels cautioning their patrons to handle the contents with care in order to prevent scalding or burning. Have you ever wondered, if these warning labels are provided for your external protection, what happens when an extremely hot or cold liquid enters the body? Our bodies are divinely calibrated to maintain a body temperature of 98.6 degrees Fahrenheit. A research study conducted at Albert Einstein College of Medicine, revealed that the 98-degree range is in perfect balance [14]. This temperature is warm enough to prevent fungal infection, but not so hot that we cannot properly maintain our metabolism. Because of this, wisdom dictates that what we eat and drink should be lower or as close as possible to this temperature.

One of the responsibilities of our red blood cells is to help regulate the body's temperature. If you're outside and the climate is very warm or if you're engaging in aerobic exercise, your blood cells will increase their flow, resulting in warmer skin and faster heat loss to help keep your body properly cooled [15]. When environmental temperatures drop, your blood flow focuses more on the internal organs deep inside the body to keep it warm. Just as the external factors of climate and exercise can affect the body, so does regularly drinking icy cold beverages.

Although this subject is not given much attention in Western medicine, traditional Chinese medicine and Ayurvedic medicine both reveal that when cold liquids are ingested and enter the stomach, the body is forced to expend greater amounts of energy to keep it balanced. This energy is needed to keep the digestive system working properly. Icy cold beverages aggravate the digestive tract, lower stomach temperature, and halt the digestion process. As cold liquid passes through the body, it causes congealing in the intestinal walls, hardening fats from food that have been eaten, making it even harder to digest properly. Digestive disorders affect 60 to 70 million people in the United States and include a number of conditions, such as: heartburn, constipation, hemorrhoids, irritable bowel syndrome, ulcers, gallstones, celiac disease (a genetic disorder in which consumption of gluten damages the intestines), and inflammatory bowel diseases including Crohn's disease, which causes ulcers to form in the gastrointestinal tract [16]. Could drinking cold liquids be one of the contributing factors yielding these high statistics? Based on these extremely high numbers, we cannot rule out the possibility of this strong correlation. Drinking extremely hot liquids can be just a detrimental.

Internally, your body is comprised of thousands of sensitive nerves, tissues, and cells. Extremely hot drinks damage sensitive nerves in your tongue, dull your taste buds and can cause you to lose your sense of taste. Hot liquids have also been shown to scar the esophagus and stomach lining. In a research study entitled, "High-temperature Beverages and Foods and Esophageal Cancer Risk - A Systematic Review," researchers cited the connection between extremely hot foods and beverages and esophageal cancer [17]. The report revealed that liquids and foods that are too hot injure esophageal cells, paving the way for esophageal cancer. Researchers concluded that letting drinks cool off from scalding temperatures to being tolerably warm or even lukewarm before swallowing is a life-saving health move.

God Always Has a Purpose

To everything there is a purpose. God designed our bodies to remain at 98.6 degrees to keep the body balanced and the daily cycle of consuming liquids that are too hot or cold creates a type of yo-yo effect that overburdens the body. The best and safest way to enjoy water and other beverages is at room temperature. To help benefit your overall health, try the following experiment. Forego cold and hot beverages and drink water at room temperature for two weeks and take note of how you feel. You should mark noticeable improvements in your health, such as improved digestion, less bloating, decreased stomach irritation, and less constipation.

Why I'm Not a Fan of Bottled Water

Not too long ago water use to be free. Today it is a multi-billion-dollar business, grossing $100 Billion annually around the globe. Countless store shelves are lined with a vast selection of the finest bottled water imports from around the world: Fiji, Italy, France, Sweden, Canada, the list goes on. In addition to the wide selection, there are also various types of water to choose from: artesian, spring, purified, sparkling, distilled, mineral, flavored, and carbonated. Bottled water has become the number one selling beverage, surpassing milk, juice, and soda [18]. Major marketing campaigns have been the driving component surrounding the increased sale of bottled water. Consumers are influenced to believe that bottled water is much safer and cleaner to drink and tastes better than regular tap water. I must admit I have enjoyed some great tasting brands of bottled water, but one day I had to ask myself: is bottled water really safer and healthier than tap water? The answer may surprise you.

How Safe Is Bottled Water?

I appreciate the fact that I receive an annual report from my public utility company, outlining the safety tests that were conducted on water that I use from the city. The report covers sanitary measures that were taken to ensure that the water is clean and safe for use and consumption. Unlike public water utility companies, bottled water companies are not required by law to provide an annual report concerning water safety. Consumers have no knowledge of where the water comes from, what is put into the water, what sanitary measures are taken to purify the water if any at all or if safety testing is conducted. The fact that bottled water companies are not required to produce or publish documentation to verify their safety and sanitary measures leaves much speculation surrounding their practices. Tap water is regulated by the Environmental Protection Agency (EPA), while bottled water is regulated by the FDA.

All drinking water must meet the same minimum standards, but EPA standards are more rigorous than what the FDA requires. For example, water treatment plants that provide tap water must be tested for contaminants multiple times a day whereas the FDA tests bottling plants only once a week [19]. Additionally, the EPA requires the disinfection of tap water, bans E. Coli and fecal coliform, tests for cryptosporidium and giardia viruses, requires that operators are trained and certified, directs certified labs for testing, and provides consumers with the right to know about contamination [20]. The FDA does not mandate any of the above standards. Comparing industry regulations confirms that companies are selling contaminated water from unknown sources to the public. On top of contaminated water, plastic bottles are comprised of cancer-causing materials such as Bisphenol-A or (BPA) [21].

> *Nearly 200 scientific studies show that exposures to low doses of BPA, particularly during prenatal development and early infancy, are associated with a wide range of adverse health effects in later life. These effects include increased risk of breast and prostate cancer, genital abnormalities in male babies, infertility in men, early puberty in girls, metabolic disorders such as insulin resistant (Type 2) diabetes and obesity, and neurobehavioral problems such as attention deficit hyperactivity disorder (ADHD). Exposures that occur before birth are particularly troubling, as the effects on the developing fetus are irreversible.*
> *Abstracts of Selected Bisphenol-A*
> *(BPA) Studies, Breast Cancer Fund*

While it is true that bottled water may taste better, ironically, it's highly toxic. While the demand for bottled water continues to increase, the impact on our financial and environmental health are also at stake.

How Much Is Bottled Water Costing Our Nation?

I was roughly spending $35 on bottled water every month, that's $420 a year. This may seem like an insignificant amount, however, if compounded over a 15-year period, $420 accumulates to $6,300. If $420 were invested into a mutual fund with an annual rate of 8 percent, you would accumulate $13,648.51. I often think about how many more people are spending this amount or more on bottled water every year. Rather than spending extra dollars on bottled water every month with no rate of return, what could you do for your family, church, or community with this extra money? On top of consumers paying their regular water bill, they are also spending extra money on overpriced contaminated water. Bottled water is being sold at a price 2,900 higher than regular tap water not including the transportation costs associated with importing and exporting bottled water [22, 23]. In 2006, the Pacific Institute estimated that:

- Producing bottles for American consumption required the equivalent of more than 17 million barrels of oil annually, not including the energy for transportation.

- Bottling water produced more than 2.5 million tons of greenhouse gases. Greenhouse gases have been shown to adversely affect the environment by altering weather patterns, causing global warming and threaten the health of vegetation around the world.

- The total amount of energy embedded in our use of bottled water can be as high as the equivalent of filling a plastic bottle with one quarter full of oil.

- It took 3 liters of water to produce 1 liter of bottled water.

Recycling is encouraged in our country, but unfortunately most people do not practice it. This results in billions of plastic water bottles accumulating in landfills every year, polluting the planet that has been entrusted to our care. Plastic bottles do not break down naturally and can take hundreds of years to decompose while releasing toxic chemicals into the ground and atmosphere.

> *Although convenient, bottled water has proven that it simply is not the most responsible choice environmentally, financially, and health-wise and must be met with more viable options.*

One of the most inexpensive, safe, and healthy alternative approaches that you can take to drinking bottled water is to invest in a quality water filter.

Alternative to Drinking Bottled Water

Investing in a quality water filter will provide you and your family with an unlimited supply of clean drinking water. Some of the most basic and common water filters brands are Pur and Britta and on average cost anywhere between twenty to forty dollars. They are both easy to install and readily snap onto to your kitchen faucet and allow you to replace the filter every 2-3 months. If you want to have clean water for your entire home, larger systems can be utilized such as the Berkey Water Filter System. Lager water filter systems require fewer filter replacement and can last for up to four years. Quality filters remove compounds found in water to include [24, 25]:

- Radon

- Pesticides

- Industrial pollutants

- Bad tastes and odors

- Parasites and bacteria

- Disinfection byproducts such as chlorine

- Heavy metals such as copper, lead, and mercury

- Pharmaceuticals including antibiotics, mood stabilizers and hormones

Not only do they remove contaminates, quality filters provide great-tasting water, and in my opinion tastes 110% better than bottled water. When shopping for a filter, ensure that it is certified by the National Sanitation Foundation and is designed to reduce contaminates in water.

Bring Your Own Bottled Water (BYOBW)

The business of bottling water has caused a dangerous ripple effect, straining the environment, health, finances, and natural resources of our nation. Individuals are becoming more conscious about these negative effects and are opting to use BPA free plastic, glass, or stainless steel refillable water bottles. Some refillable water bottles have filters attached to them or you can purchase portable filters that can be easily placed inside of the water bottle allowing you to have access to clean water wherever you go. Quality refillable water bottles are relatively inexpensive and can be purchased for under fifteen dollars and offer a sound solution towards healthier living.

There's Healing in the Water

What would your health look like if you began drinking water on a regular basis? How would you feel? If you truly want to begin improving your health, drinking water every day is one of the most important keys that you can incorporate into your lifestyle. Many of your bodily functions may simply be out of sync because they are lacking nutrients that only water can provide. When God created water, He designed it to be liquid energy for the body, replenishing, and infusing every blood cell with life and strength. Even though American culture promotes consuming other drinks over plain water, we must take the time to pause and seriously consider the repercussions that are resulting from not drinking enough water. Water is God's miracle liquid. It's time to embrace and begin enjoying this perfectly designed drink, for truly, blessings, and healing are in the water.

> *O taste and see that the Lord [our God] is good! Blessed (happy, fortunate, to be envied) is the man who trusts and takes refuge in Him.*
>
> *Psalms 34:8*

Key # 4 - Drink clean filtered water to keep the body hydrated and operating at optimal levels

Healthy Ways to Rock Your Body Naturally with Water

- Learn to listen to your body. Instead of reaching for a sugar-sweetened drink, give your body what it needs by drinking clean filtered tap water.

- Purchase a quality water filter to use at home and/or your job. You can find out which brand is best for you by visiting www.waterfiltercomparisons.com. You can also visit the National Sanitation Foundation at http://info.nsf.org/Certified/dwtu/ to find information about certified water filters.

- Commit to increase your daily intake of water. If you're just starting out, trying drinking one cup of water 30 minutes before breakfast, 30 minutes before lunch and 30 minutes before dinner (before 7 p.m.). This will help you to get into the habit of drinking water regularly throughout the day and will also aid in proper digestion.

- Add fun and variety to your water by infusing fresh or frozen fruit or a splash of 100% fruit juice such as blueberry, apple, cherry, or pomegranate.

- Keep your body balanced by drinking water at room temperature. This will help to maintain the body's natural temperature range of 98.6 degrees.

- Get into the habit of drinking beverages warm and not scalding hot. This practice will prevent damaging sensitive body tissue and healthy cells.

- Turn your water into a delicious meal by making warm healing soups and broths. Add organic non-GMO vegetables to include carrots, parsley, broccoli, onions, spinach, or kale.

- Juicing fresh fruits and vegetables is a great way to hydrate your body with water. Not only do fruits and vegetables contain an abundance of water they also contain vital nutrients to detox and feed your blood cells.

- Visit your city's local website to view an online copy of your annual water report. The report will provide a detailed description of what sanitary types of tests were conducted, as well as the results. If you cannot access the report online, call your municipality's main office to request an electronic copy to be sent to you via e-mail.

- Invest the money that you spend on bottled water in a mutual fund with a rate of return of 8% or more. To see your potential savings, use a compound interest calculator by using the Google search engine.

- Bring Your Own Bottled Water (BYOBW). Carry your own refillable water bottle. Go to my web site at rockyourworldnaturally.com and click on the book link and go to resources to find affordable quality bottles.

Key # 5

Incorporate Essential Oils
Into Your World Daily

[Essential Oil / the most vital and
natural elements of a plant's fragrance]

Fruit trees of all kinds will grow on both banks of the river.
Their leaves will not wither, nor will their fruit fail.
Every month they will bear fruit, because the
water from the sanctuary flows to them.
Their fruit will serve for food and
their leaves for healing.

Ezekiel 47:12

You shall make of these a holy anointing oil, a perfume mixture, the work of a perfumer; it shall be a holy anointing oil.
Exodus 30:25

Chapter 7

Why Essential Oils Are a Must in Your World

Our First Medicine

F rom Genesis to Revelations, just about every book in the bible speaks about plant life and their diverse properties. After God finished creating the earth, He looked upon all that He made and said that it was good and very good.

> *And God saw everything that he had made, and behold, it was very good. And there was evening and there was morning, the sixth day.*
>
> *Genesis 1:31*

Animals roamed the earth freely, aquatic life teemed in the seas and oceans, birds inhabited the sky, and Adam and Eve dwelled peaceably in the Garden of Eden—a tranquil paradise that was abundantly populated with plant life. Everything in God's creation was designed with a distinct purpose. When God finished His work on the sixth day, all that we needed to live comfortably in the earth was provided. Plant life was not only created to adorn the earth with beauty, but plants provided habitation and food for animals and shelter, food, clothing, and medicine for humans.

> *And God said, "Let the earth sprout vegetation, plants yielding seed, and fruit trees bearing fruit in which is their seed, each according to its kind, on the earth." And it was so.*
>
> *Genesis 1:11*

> *Through the middle of the street of the city; also, on either side of the river, the tree of life with its twelve kinds of fruit, yielding its fruit each month. The leaves of the tree were for the healing of the nations.*
>
> *Revelations 22:2*

When God created our bodies, He formed us from the dust of the earth. Therefore, our physical composition is organic and consists of elements found in the earth such as oxygen, carbon, hydrogen, nitrogen, calcium, and phosphorus. Because of this fact, our bodies respond positively and work in perfect agreement with earth derived, plant-based healing approaches. Although plant-based healing methodologies are not widely accepted or readily used within conventional settings, their use and effectiveness is grabbing the attention of individuals seeking alternatives to taking prescription medication. Essential Oils provide plant-based healing that is natural, safe, highly effective, and biblically centered. These miraculous oils were created to keep the body aligned, healed, and balanced.

What Are Essential Oils?

Essential Oils have always been a part of God's creation and are referenced in the bible over 600 times [1]. Essential Oils are called essential because they contain the most vital and natural elements of plant life and are derived from bark, trees, flowers, leaves, fruit, seeds, or roots [2]. The liquid essence extracted from these plants is not actually oil, but has an oil-like appearance, thus the name Essential Oils. In ancient times, these plant extractions came in various forms to include tree gum, incense, spices, perfume, resin, and oil. Today, the primary means of extracting Essential Oils is through the process of steam distillation. When captured, these plant essences are highly concentrated, intensely aromatic, and contain a number of remarkable healing properties.

> *Through steam distillation, plant material is placed in an extraction chamber and then steam (produced by boiling water in another chamber) is released into the bottom of the extraction chamber where the plant material is. As the steam passes through the plant material, both the steam and the Essential Oil rise to the top. The steam and Essential Oil are directed to another chamber where they are allowed to cool. As the oil and steam mixture cools, the essential oil rises to the top of the chamber while the water stays at the bottom. Through this process, the Essential Oil can then be easily separated from the water.*
> *Modern Essentials A Contemporary Guide to the Therapeutic Use of Essential Oils*

Essential Oils and the Bible

In the bible, Essential Oils were recorded as being used by Moses, priests, and kings, and by people from all different walks of life. In the book of Leviticus, the Levite priests were responsible for incorporating Essential Oils into everyday living and used them during times of worship, celebration, prayer, cleansing, healing, burial, fasting, and consecration.

> *And Jacob rose up early in the morning, and took the stone that he had put [for] his pillows, and set it up [for] a pillar, and poured oil upon the top of it.*
> *Genesis 28:18*

> *Then the LORD said to Moses, "take for yourself spices, stacte and onycha and galbanum, spices with*

pure frankincense; there shall be an equal part of each. With it you shall make incense, a perfume, the work of a perfumer, salted, pure, and holy. You shall beat some of it very fine, and put part of it before the testimony in the tent of meeting where I will meet with you; it shall be most holy to you. The incense which you shall make, you shall not make in the same proportions for yourselves; it shall be holy to you for the LORD."

Exodus 30:34-37

Then Moses took the anointing oil and anointed the tabernacle and everything in it, and so consecrated them.

Leviticus 8:10

And the priest shall take some of the log of oil, and pour it into the palm of his own left hand: and the priest shall dip his right finger in the oil that is in his left hand, and shall sprinkle of the oil with his finger seven times before the LORD: and of the rest of the oil that is in his hand shall the priest put upon the tip of the right ear of him that is to be cleansed, and upon the thumb of his right hand, and upon the great toe of his right foot, upon the blood of the trespass offering: and the remnant of the oil that is in the priest's hand he shall pour upon the head of him that is to be cleansed: and the priest shall make an atonement for him before the LORD.

Leviticus 14:15-18

Then Samuel took a vial of oil, and poured [it] upon his head, and kissed him, and said, [Is it] not because the LORD hath anointed thee [to be] captain over his inheritance?

I Samuel 10:1

And behold, a woman of the city, who was a sinner, when she learned that he was reclining at table in the Pharisee's house, brought an alabaster flask of ointment, and standing behind him at his feet, weeping, she began to wet his feet with her tears and wiped them with the hair of her head and kissed his feet and anointed them with the ointment.

Luke 7:37-40

Essential Oils were even used in royal beauty regiments. When Queen Esther was chosen to stand before King Ahasuerus, she spent one full year undergoing beauty treatments that included the Essential Oil myrrh, sweet spices, and perfumes. These extracts moisturized the skin and also promoted physical healing and internal cleansing.

Now when the turn of each maiden came to go in to King Ahasuerus, after the regulations for the women had been carried out for twelve months—since this was the regular period for their beauty treatments, six months with oil of myrrh and six months with sweet spices and perfumes and the things for the purifying of the women.

Esther 2:12

At Jesus' birth, the wise men brought Him gifts of frankincense, myrrh, and gold. Frankincense and myrrh were aromatic resins derived from trees and were commonly used for incense and perfumes. Throughout the Old Testament, priests regularly used frankincense during times of worship and sacrifice, symbolizing holiness and righteousness. The gift of frankincense was symbolic of Jesus being our High Priest, and also signified the ultimate holy righteous sacrifice of Jesus Christ. The gift of myrrh symbolized the death that Jesus was to endure on the cross. Though His assignment was filled with great bitterness and suffering, His death purchased our glorious salvation.

143

> *And they tried to give Him wine mixed with myrrh; but*
> *He did not take it.*
>
> *Mark 15:23*

In addition to the Bible, other ancient writings further denote how various cultures used these oils. Like Queen Esther, Egyptian historians documented Cleopatra as regularly using Essential Oils as part of her beauty treatments [3]. The Romans used Essential Oils and considered them to be a mark of superiority representing prosperity and abundance. In China, Egypt, India, and Greece, Essential Oils were commonly used for perfume and spiritual, therapeutic, hygienic, and ritualistic purposes [4]. The Corpus Hippocraticum, a recorded collection of medicinal works, contains hundreds of writings from the Greek physician Hippocrates, further authenticating the effectiveness of aromatic plant extracts used to naturally heal the body [5]. There are over a dozen Essential Oils mentioned in the bible, with each one possessing a specific healing property and spiritual significance. Some of the most commonly used Essential Oils were cinnamon, calamus, hyssop, cedar wood, frankincense, myrrh, and spikenard [6].

Essential Oil	Healing Properties/Uses	Spiritual Significance
Hyssop	Digestive Issues, Asthma, Urinary Tract Infections, Improve Circulation, Bruises, Frostbite, Colic, Liver Problems, Poor Circulation, HIV/AIDS Treatment.	Used during purification ceremonies and for internal cleansing. Represents the power and inner working of the Holy Spirit to bring deliverance, cleansing, forgiveness and healing. Exodus 12:22, Psalms 51.
Myrrh	Skin Allergies, Gum Disease, Infection, Skin Wounds or Skin Problems, Supports the Immune System, Arthritis Pain, Hemorrhoids, Wounds, Abrasions, Menstrual Flow, Cancer, Leprosy, Syphilis, Lung Congestion, Boils, Colds and Indigestion.	Symbolizes dying to self. Though Jesus' death was filled with great bitterness and suffering, He died to himself in order to purchase our glorious salvation. Queen Esther sacrificed her will in order to save the Jewish nation. Mark 15:23, Esther 2:12.

Cinnamon	Antibacterial, Antifungal, Diabetes, Mold, Premature Ejaculation, Respiratory Infection, Warming, Reduces Menstrual Pain, Relieves Arthritis and Cramps.	Signifies God's desire to receive the sweet aroma of holy and fragrant worship from His children. It is also a symbol of God's love being poured out upon His church. Exodus 30:23, Solomon 4:13-15.
Calamus	Gastrointestinal (GI) Problems Including Ulcers, Inflammation of the Stomach Lining, Upset Stomach, Loss of Appetite (Anorexia), Sedative to Calm Nerves, Rheumatoid Arthritis and Stroke.	As Believers, we have been bought with a price, the Blood of Jesus. In the scriptures, this spice is representative of the call for every Christian to live a life that is consecrated and separated completely to the Lord Jesus Christ. Exodus 30:23, Ezekiel 27:19, Solomon 4:14.
Cassia	Flatulence, Muscle and Stomach Spasms, Nausea, Diarrhea, Erectile Dysfunction, Menopausal Symptoms, Kidney Disorders, High Blood Pressure, Blood Purifier and Cancer.	Cassia translated in Hebrew is *"qiddah"* meaning to strip off. Symbolic of putting off the old man and putting on the new man in Christ. Old things have passed away and all things are new. Exodus 30:24, Psalms 45:8, 2 Corinthians 5:17.
Juniper	Urinary Tract Infections, Kidney and Bladder Stones, Diabetes, Cancer, Snakebites, Skin Wounds, Joint and Muscle Pain, Bronchitis, Upset Stomach, and Bloating.	Juniper trees were often used for shelter from the elements and for fuel. We can rest assured that through every phase of life, God meets every one of our needs. He is our covering and provides us with spiritual and natural shelter. The fire of His Holy Spirit burns within us and is the fuel that helps us to live a victorious Christian life. Philippians 4:19, I Kings 19:4-5, Job 30:4, Psalms 120:4.

Pine	Antibacterial, Disinfectant, Antiseptic, Natural Deodorizer, Influenza, Herpes Simplex Type 1 & 2, E. Coli, Candida Albicans, Lower Respiratory Tract Swelling, Inflammation, Cold, Cough, Bronchitis, Fevers, Blood Pressure, Stuffy Nose, Muscle Pain and Nerve Pain.	Pine is translated as *"shemen"* in the Hebrew meaning fat oil, representative of God's anointing, fruitfulness, and prosperity. It was also known as the wild olive tree, symbolic of the Christian life. As the wild olive tree, we have been engrafted into the True Olive Tree, Christ, and are now able to partake of His goodness and mercy. Isaiah 4:19, Isaiah 60:13, Nehemiah 8:15, Romans 11:16-24.
Cedar wood	Antifungal, Disinfectant, Household Cleaning, Skin Care, Alopecia (Hair Loss) and Insect Repellent.	Used during cleansing and purification ceremonies by priests along with a scarlet thread and hyssop signifying that only through the blood of Jesus can we receive cleansing and forgiveness of sins. This stately tree was also referred to as the glory of Israel, symbolic of God's power, peace and love for His people. Leviticus 14:4-6, Leviticus 14:51-52 Numbers 24:6, I Kings 6:9-10, I Kings 7:2-7.
Frankincense	Osteoarthritis, Rheumatoid Arthritis, Joint Pain, Bursitis, Tendonitis, Ulcerative Colitis, Abdominal Pain, Hay Fever, Sore Throat, Syphilis, Menstruation, Pimples and Cancer.	Used regularly during times of worship and sacrifice, symbolizing holiness and righteousness. The Magi brought Frankincense as a gift at Jesus' birth acknowledging Him as our King, High Priest and the ultimate holy sacrifice. He was righteous in all of His ways, and selflessly gave His life for sinful mankind. Exodus 30:34-37, Matthew 1:11.

Myrtle	Antifungal, Antibacterial, Treating Lung Infections, Bronchitis, Whooping Cough, Tuberculosis, Bladder Conditions, Diarrhea and Worms.	Instead of the thorn shall come up the fir-tree, and instead of the brier shall come up the myrtle-tree, a prophetic picture of God's grace, mercy and promised blessings. Nehemiah 8:15, Zechariah 1:8,10,11, Isaiah 41:18-20, Isaiah 55:13.
Galbanum	Skin Wounds, Digestive Problems, Flatulence, Poor Appetite, Cough and Spasms.	Galbanum comes from the Hebrew word *"chelbanah or khelbnah"* meaning *"fatness."* As we draw closer to God in worship, He will bless us in body, soul and spirit with His fatness or prosperity, goodness and abundance. Exodus 30:34, Genesis 27:28, Proverbs 13:4.
Aloes (Sandalwood)	Common Cold, Cough, Bronchitis, Fever, Sore Mouth and Throat, Urinary Tract Infection, Liver Disease, Gallbladder Problems, Heatstroke, Headache, Conditions of the Heart and Blood Vessels (Cardiovascular Disease).	After the Crucifixion of Jesus, this spice was used to prepare Jesus' physical body for burial, symbolizing great love, honor and respect. These same themes are present when Aloes are mentioned throughout the Bible. John 19:39, Solomon 4:14, Psalms 45:8, Numbers 24:6.
Rose of Sharon	Stomach Irritation, Disorders of Circulation, Laxative, Diuretic, Upper Respiratory Tract Pain and Swelling, Heart and Nerve Diseases, Loss of Appetite, Colds, Fluid Retention.	The bible depicts Jesus as the Rose of Sharon. A rose given to His children, a beautiful expression of God's undying love for the church. As God's presence fills our lives, in return we become a sweet fragrance to God and the world. Solomon 1:17, Solomon 2:1.

| Spikenard | Skin Disease Treatment, Coughs, Asthma, Arthritis, Loosen Congestion, Boost Tissue Regrowth and Promotes Sweating. | Prophetically spoken of by king Solomon, this expensive and highly prized oil was lavishly poured out upon Jesus prior to His Crucifixion. When translated in the Greek it means pure, representing Jesus as the perfect Lamb of God. Jesus now sits at the right hand of the Father in heaven and receives our worship as the fragrance of spikenard, pleasing and acceptable unto Him. Solomon 1:12, Solomon 4:13-14, Mark 14:3, John 12:3-5. |

The Importance of Using Quality Essential Oils

Essential Oils contain powerful healing properties, but not all oils are created equal. Many Essential Oils on the market contain little to no health value and can even be toxic to your health. If you choose to use Essential Oils, ensure that they are 100% pure Certified Therapeutic Grade Essential Oils. Therapeutic grade oils contain the most potent and highest grade of plant oil and possess the greatest healing properties.

Essential Oils are extremely concentrated and highly medicinal. Because they are natural medicine, you should consult a trained and experienced Certified Aromatherapist, Certified Herbalist, physician or naturopathic practitioner who is knowledgeable about Essential Oils before using them. This can help determine if you will have any reactions to the oil, especially if you are taking prescription medications. When applied to the skin, Essential Oils must always be mixed with organic carrier oils to dilute the oil such as coconut, sweet almond, avocado, grapeseed, jojoba, and olive. These are known as carrier oils because they help to carry the Essential Oils onto the skin [7]. A small percentage of individuals experience reactions such as skin irritation or allergies with skin application. Improper ingestion of Certified Therapeutic Essential Oils can result in vomiting, seizures, or can even death [8]. There are also Food Grade Essential Oils that can be safely ingested and used for cooking.

Essential Oils should only be used based on your bio-individuality and specific health needs to reap the maximum health benefits.

When used properly, Essential Oils have the natural ability to produce healing and wholeness within the body at the cellular level. Because the health of our blood is crucial to the prevention of disease, using Essential Oils on a regular basis is vital to experiencing and maintaining extraordinary health.

How Do They Work?

The two primary ways that Essential Oils enter the body are through the nose (inhalation/breathing) and the skin (absorption through massage). The nose is one of our most powerful sense organs and is connected to our limbic system. The limbic system supports a variety of functions to include memory, behavior, emotions, motivation, hormone levels, and stress reactions. One of the easiest ways to experience the health benefits of Essential Oils is by using a diffuser. A diffuser releases a fine mist into the air, making it easy to inhale the oil. When diffused, Essential Oils purify the air, remove toxins, destroy mold, inhibit bacterial growth, increase atmospheric oxygen and remove metallic particles. The scriptures remind us that God takes great pleasure in fragrant smells, especially when we offer our heartfelt worship up to Him.

May my prayer be set before you like incense; may the lifting up of my hands be like the evening sacrifice.
Psalms 141:2

And walk in love, just as Christ also loved you and gave Himself up for us, an offering and a sacrifice to God as a fragrant aroma.
Ephesians 5:2

*Then Aaron's sons shall offer it up in smoke on the altar on
the burnt offering, which is on the wood that is on the fire;
it is an offering by fire of a soothing aroma to the Lord.*
Leviticus 3:5

Because we are made in the likeness and image of our Father, we are no different. The sense of smell is very powerful and when our bodies come in contact with a specific fragrance it responds. For instance, the effervescent fragrance of fresh lemons has been known to boost your mood and brighten your spirits. Or have your ever smelled an aroma that triggered a pleasant memory? This is certainly true when cooking a favorite family recipe. These are both examples of how God designed our sense of smell to work hand-in-hand with our limbic system. Research has shown that when aroma and the sense of smell merge, they work in unity, significantly influencing moods, memory recall and bodily responses such as heart rate, respiration, hormone levels, and stress reactions [10]. When inhaled, Essential Oils release potent healing properties into the bloodstream that increase energy levels, heal the body, enhance mood and promote relaxation.

Essential Oils and Your Bloodstream

As we've seen, toxins enter the bloodstream by eating unhealthy food, from our environment and through poor lifestyle habits. If toxic waste continues to build up in our system, our red blood cells become damaged and we get sick. When absorbed through the skin or inhaled through the nose, Essential Oils enter the bloodstream, naturally metabolize like other nutrients and heal the body at the cellular level. This form of plant-based healing was uniquely designed to work in unity with our bloodstream. This is the major difference between plant-based healing and prescription medications.

Presently, most illnesses are treated with pharmaceutical drugs composed of inorganic compounds that the human body cannot recognize, properly absorb or digest, nor do they heal our blood cells. More often than not, toxins from these compounds cause several harmful side-effects, complicating health issues even further. If you've watched or listened to the latest pharmaceutical advertisements and the possible side-effects that can stem from taking a specific prescription it's quite alarming. I can't help but cringe when an advertisement for a new medication is offered to the population [10].

> *In 2012, the pharmaceutical industry spent more than $27 billion marketing drugs over the television, internet and radio. When broken down, this equates to more than $24 billion being spent on marketing to physicians and over $3 billion to individuals, heavily influencing doctors and patients to prescribe and consume prescription drugs. The United States is one of only two countries in the world that allows direct drug advertising to consumers; the other is New Zealand.*

Dollars Over Health

Each advertisement always seems to start out the same. A man or woman with a soothing voice and soft music in the background talks about all of the amazing benefits of the medication and then, towards the end of the advertisement, you hear things like: this medication may cause heart attacks, seizures, high blood pressure, insomnia, sleepwalking, depression, migraine headaches, hallucinations, or sudden death, use at your own risk. Just listening to this type of advertisement could cause anyone's anxiety level to rise. Prescription medications are supposed to help you feel better, and yet millions of Americans are walking through life in a state of toxic overload as a result of using ineffective prescription medications. Advertisements contribute to the US' global pharmaceutical industry, which earns over $300 billion annually [11].

The pharmaceutical industry is controlled by ten of the largest drug companies, with several of them earning over $10 billion a year. Rather than spending most of the revenue earned from these sales on the research and development of pharmaceuticals, one-third is spent on marketing and advertisements. The pharmaceutical industry has become a system that is driven by greed, with no genuine regard for the recovery of individual health. The lack of adequate research and development for prescription drugs has become one of the leading causes of injury death in the United States.

The Straight Facts About Prescription Medications

Reports from the Centers for Disease Control and Prevention reveal that deaths from prescription drug overdose have risen steadily over the past two decades and have become the leading cause of injury death in the United States. Every day in the United States, 114 people die as a result of prescription drug overdose, and another 6,748 are treated in emergency departments for the misuse or abuse of prescription drugs. Prescription drugs cause nearly nine out of ten deaths by poisoning and prescription drug overdose was the leading cause of injury death in 2012. Among people 25 to 64 years old, overdose caused more deaths than motor vehicle traffic crashes. Among children under age 6, pharmaceuticals account for about 40% of all exposures reported to poison centers [12.]

The United States is in the midst of a prescription painkiller overdose epidemic. Since 1999, the amount of prescription painkillers prescribed and sold in the U.S. has nearly quadrupled, yet there has not been an overall change in the amount of pain that Americans report. Over prescribing leads to more abuse and more overdose deaths.
Centers for Disease Control and Prevention

These staggering statistics reveal that there is an all-out assault on our health. Now is the time to take bold spiritual and natural approaches to guard our divine health. Far too many lives are ending before their destiny has been fulfilled as a result of using ineffective prescription drugs. Synthetic medications do provide some form of temporary relief; however, the methods in place continually prove that prescription medication is not the most effective way to treat illnesses. As the Apostle Paul shares in I Corinthians 12:31, God has a better or more excellent way.

The weapons we fight with are not the weapons of the world. On the contrary, they have divine power to demolish strongholds.
2 Corinthians 10:4

The More Excellent Way

Although not approved by the FDA, studies consistently reveal that Essential Oils have been used to effectively treat a wide variety of diseases, such as cancer, skin disorders, asthma, Traumatic Brain Injury, depression, arthritis, HIV/AIDS, anxiety, menopause, coma recovery, sexual dysfunction, ADD/ADHD, autoimmune diseases, bronchitis, strokes, and paralysis [13, 14]. Essential Oils are proving to be so successful in treating diseases that a new nationwide government survey confirms that more than one-third of adults in the U.S. are using plant-based or herbal healing remedies [15]. Individuals are discovering the benefits of plant-based treatments as they are proving to be more cost-effective, easily absorb into the bloodstream with no pills to take, achieve long-term healing results and do not have the dangerous side-effects associated with most prescription medications. Their effectiveness is even gaining traction within the healthcare system.

Hospitals Are Beginning to Follow God's Original Blueprint

In 2014, The Cleveland Clinic, one of the country's top hospitals, opened one of the first hospital-based herbal clinics in the United States, providing their patients with more natural and holistic approaches to health that address prevention and treatment of chronic disease. They are establishing what could be considered the national model for integrating plant-based clinics into U.S. hospitals. Herbalist at The Cleveland Clinic prescribe plant blends based on research which has shown to help manage diabetes, decrease cold/flu symptoms, manage chronic pain, increase energy, improve breathing, digestion, sleep, and menopausal symptoms, and help address menstrual cycles if infertility is an issue [16]. It is more than promising and speaks volumes to see alternative approaches to healthcare being implemented. This has always been God's original blueprint for our health.

Breaking Away from the American Way

In America, our culture is inundated with advertisements that readily encourage the use of prescription medications. Unfortunately, this has become the norm. During a routine doctor's visit, my physician was shocked to discover that I was not taking any medications. She looked at me and said, "Good, keep it this way. Stay off of medications." I thought, if you are telling me to stay off of medications, why are so many physicians prescribing medications to patients' day in and day out?

Like so many others, I've been there. When I was taking a lot of medication, I never remember feeling completely well. I trusted that what I was taking was beneficial to my health and never questioned the short-term or long-term effects of medication on my body. I did not fully understand how it impacted the health of my blood cells. Many individuals are in this same position and are being prescribed medication after medication, without considering the damaging long-term effects of synthetic substances on the human body. When I was introduced to Essential Oils over a decade ago, I was so blessed by the results that I cannot imagine living without them.

We Must Change Our Approach

As people of faith, our first approach to address any kind of illness should always begin with prayer. Prayer is necessary to seek God's guidance, wisdom, and direction.

> *Is anyone among you sick? Let them call the elders of the church to pray over them and anoint them with oil in the name of the Lord. And the prayer offered in faith will make the sick person well; the Lord will raise them up. If they have sinned, they will be forgiven. Therefore, confess your sins to each other and pray for each other so that you may be healed. The prayer of a righteous person is powerful and effective.*
>
> *James 5:14-16*

God has a number of different avenues that He can use to bring about our physical healing. He can perform a supernatural miracle through the prayer of faith or He can work through a health professional or He may require us to add works to our faith. Most of the time, He wants us to add works to our faith so that we can reap the health benefits of our diligent efforts. Many times, when we seek God for healing, our faith is strong and we believe that He can heal and will heal us, however, outside of our faith, we are not taking any purposeful actions to possess and walk in our healing.

> *In the same way, faith by itself, if it is not accompanied by action, is dead.*
>
> *James 2:17*

God has already given us everything that we need that pertains to life and godliness, and one of those things is Essential Oils. Instead of automatically reverting to using a synthetic medication, consider using an Essential Oil. Please understand that I am not advising you to stop using your current medication. To do so without integrating an alternative method without sound medical advice is dangerous. What I am offering is an alternative approach that can help to gradually free you up from depending on and taking prescription medications, and instead embrace a lasting and naturally healing approach. Many people have been conditioned to believe that prescription drugs are the only way to treat their illnesses. The striking statistics on prescription drugs clearly proves that this is not true. The truth is that God wants us to walk and live in His promise of health. Knowing the truth about Essential Oils is one of the keys that can aid in releasing us from the bondage of sickness and disease.

> *Beloved, I pray that you may prosper in every way and [that your body] may keep well, even as [I know] your soul keeps well.*
>
> *3 John 2*

Much like our eating, Christians have separated our spiritually from our physical health. God has always purposed our spirit, soul, and body to function in one accord.

May God himself, the God of peace, sanctify you through and through. May your whole spirit, soul and body be kept blameless at the coming of our Lord Jesus Christ.
I Thessalonians 5:23

Thus says the LORD, "Stand by the ways and see and ask for the ancient paths, Where the good way is, and walk in it; and you will find rest for your souls. But they said, 'We will not walk in it."
Jeremiah 6:16

As the Body of Christ, we must return to God's simplistic natural pathways to health and healing through Essential Oils. We can rest assured that God's ways are always good and will never fail us. When we make a genuine effort to use this divine key, we will rise to new levels of health and discover the wonderful rest that God has always intended for His children.

Key # 5 - Incorporate Essential Oils Into Your World Daily

Healthy Ways to Rock Your World Naturally with Essential Oils

- Locate an experienced Certified Aromatherapist, Certified Herbalist, physician, or naturopathic practitioner who is knowledgeable about Essential Oils in your area before using them medicinally. They can help determine which Essential Oils are best for your health needs.

- For rest & relaxation common Essential Oils that are used are Lavender, Bergamont, Rose, Orange, Chamomile, and Ylang Ylang.

- Diffuse lavender oil to help you feel calm just before bed. Place a drop or two of oil on your pillow for a soothing effect. Make a spray by using 5-7 drops of oil with 1 ounce of filtered water and spray lightly into the air, on your pillows and sheets.

- To boost your energy levels common Essential Oils that may be used are Peppermint, Eucalyptus, Lemon, Wintergreen, and Thyme.

- Diffuse an invigorating oil first thing in the morning. Consider setting your diffuser 10 minutes before your alarm clock goes off to awaken the body naturally.

- Place a few drops of Eucalyptus Oil on the shower wall or shower floor for an aromatherapy experience.

- Diffuse Essential Oil in your workout area at home 10 minutes before getting started.

- Common Essential Oils that may be used to clean your house are Eucalyptus, Lemon, Melaleuca, Cinnamon, and Peppermint.

- Mix 1 cup of baking soda with 20-30 drops of Eucalyptus Oil and let it sit overnight. Sprinkle lightly over carpet and let sit for 15 minutes and vacuum.

- Put a few drops of Lemon and Eucalyptus Oil on a dust cloth to wipe down wooden furniture.

- Place a few drops of Lemon Oil in your dishwater for squeaky clean dishes.

- For prayer and meditation common Essential Oils that may be used are Frankincense, Rose, Bergamont, and Ylang Ylang. Diffuse one of these oils in a quiet place 15 minutes before reading your Bible and during times of prayer or while meditating on the scriptures. Essential Oils are a gift from God and contain no "special powers." The oils help to focus our attention on God's holy presence and create an atmosphere for deep spiritual awareness.

Key # 6

*Remember the Sabbath...rest for
the spirit, soul and body*

*[Sabbath / to stop, to cease, to rest
completely from work or labor]*

*Earnestly remember the Sabbath day,
to keep it holy, withdrawn from
[all labor] common employment
and dedicated to God.*

Exodus 20:8

And Jesus said unto them, "the Sabbath was made for man and not man for the Sabbath, therefore the son of man is Lord also of the Sabbath" Mark 2:27-28

Chapter 8

Remember the Sabbath

———————————————————

The Earth's axis is an invisible line that runs through the north and south poles around which the Earth spins. Our Creator tilted the Earth's axis at the exact degree, keeping our world, universe, and all of creation in perfect alignment. Scientific studies have shown that if the Earth's axis was not perfectly titled, the result would be total chaos. There would be no variation in the duration of daylight throughout the year, there would be no seasons, and agriculture would be affected to the point of no growing season, familiar annual cycles that animals exhibit, such as migration, food storage, mating, and hibernation, might change or cease to exist [1]. Life as we know it on Planet Earth would be disastrous.

Much like the earth, every individual possesses a personal axis, an invisible and internal spiritual place that when properly aligned with God brings rest, peace, and balance into our daily lives. In this chapter, we will explore the meaning of the Sabbath, why God created the Sabbath, and how you can use this special key to unlock inner-peace and freedom that will release you from the busyness of our society that all-too-often seems to leave us spinning out of control.

The Sabbath

When I speak to Christians and non-Christians about the Sabbath, the conversation usually does not go beyond the discussion of weekly worship. Should individuals attend church services on Saturday or Sunday? Some people say that spending time and fellowshipping with God every day is what counts and that the Sabbath was under the Old Testament law and does not apply to Christians today. Others believe that as long as you attend church services during the week or as long as you attend church on Sunday, this is observing the Sabbath. Some denominations were formed out of the belief that Christians should attend church on Saturday.

I have had the opportunity to worship with Messianic Jewish and Seventh-Day Adventist friends on Saturday. Personally, I attend church on Sunday. And there have also been times that my church has held our main worship services on Saturday. From my personal experience and perspective, there doesn't seem to be much difference concerning the main day that you choose to attend church. With all of these differences of opinion, understanding the true meaning of the Sabbath can become quite clouded. To obtain clarity, a review of the scriptures is necessary to fully comprehend how the Sabbath came about, why God created it, and how it applies to Christians and our health.

History of the Sabbath

The Sabbath is first mentioned in Exodus 16, right after God delivered the children of Israel from the bonds of Egyptian slavery. For 400 years, they were mercilessly oppressed, forced to work incessantly day in and day out under the rule of harsh taskmasters. Generations of husbands, wives, and children, were all too acquainted with the mortar, brick, and straw used to build structures to support a pagan nation. During this time in history, their hard labor catapulted Egypt into being the world's number one Superpower; a nation that boasted of its rich resources, strong government and irrefutable mastery of mathematics, arts, and the sciences. No nation could come close to Egyptian rule and in fact their empire seemed unstoppable. The drudgery of slavery had reached a crescendo loud enough to be heard in the heavens, causing the God of all Ages to respond to the children of Israel's cry.

> *Now, behold, the cry of the sons of Israel has come to*
> *Me; furthermore, I have seen the oppression with which*
> *the Egyptians are oppressing them.*
>
> *Exodus 3:9*

God miraculously used His servant Moses to deliver His children from Pharos wicked grip. After ten devastating plagues, the Egyptian nation was humbly brought down to its knees, acknowledging, and submitting to the One true God, letting Israel go so that they could worship and serve Him. God's children would now experience living a new life, one much different than the one they had known under the yoke of 400 years of slavery. God had to teach them how He wanted them to live by providing new laws that would serve to bless Israel and honor Him.

Under the old Egyptian regime, the children of Israel were accustomed to working relentlessly, leaving no time to connect with God. God provided a remedy to this problem by making room for His children to care for their spirit, soul and body by instituting the Sabbath, one of God's highest forms of self-care. God told Israel to work for six days and to reserve one day out of the week to give themselves over completely to rest. A day that would be specifically marked and separated from all others. This was so significant to God that He made it the fourth law of the Ten Commandments.

> *[Earnestly] remember the Sabbath day, to keep it holy*
> *(withdrawn from common employment and dedicated to*
> *God). Six days you shall labor and do all your work, But*
> *the seventh day is a Sabbath to the Lord your God; in it*
> *you shall not do any work, you, or your son, your*
> *daughter, your manservant, your maidservant, your*
> *domestic animals, or the sojourner within your gates. For*
> *in six days the Lord made the heavens and the earth, the*
> *sea, and all that is in them, and rested the seventh*

*day. That is why the Lord blessed the Sabbath day and
hallowed it [set it apart for His purposes].*

Exodus 20:8-11

Christians and the Sabbath

While many individuals only equate the Sabbath as being a day of worship, this is only a part of it. Clearly the scriptures explain that it is a day of rest from all laborious tasks to worship and honor God. Since this is the case, how does the Sabbath relate to Christians today? In the book of Galatians, the Apostle Paul gives godly counsel to the church regarding the observation of days, months, seasons, and years, revealing that under the new covenant, Christians are not bound to observing such things.

*You are trying to earn favor with God by observing certain
days or months or seasons or years.*

Galatians 4:10

At this particular time, there were many false teachers among the Galatians that forced them to observe certain days of the month, seasons, and years because they believed that it would draw them closer to God on a spiritual level. In all actuality, all this did was bring them into bondage and not into a personal relationship with God, directing their attention on what they could achieve, rather than focusing on what Jesus did. Jesus' death, burial, and resurrection, liberated Christians from living under any form of bondage. The scriptures remind us, whom the Son sets free, is truly free indeed. Paul expounds on this even further in the book of Colossians by providing guidance concerning the Sabbath.

*Therefore, do not let anyone judge you by what you eat or
drink, or with regard to a religious festival, a New Moon
celebration or a Sabbath day: which are a shadow of the*

things that were to come; the reality, however, is found in Christ.

Colossians 2:16-17

From the scriptures, we glean two evident truths. First, under the law, God created the Sabbath for His children as a day of rest and worship that is specifically set apart for Him. Secondly, under the New Testament Covenant, Christians are not bound by the legality of the law to observe the Sabbath, however there are many God-centered philosophies within the Sabbath that can be applied to our faith today.

Our Nation is Spinning Out of Control

Over the past 30 years, there has been a drastic shift concerning the American way of life. Unfortunately, and to our demise, our society has become one that is driven by achieving high productivity and high profits, overruling the need to rest from physical labor. We live in an era where 24/7 operations have become the norm. Much like the children of Israel, people in and out of the church are enslaved to never-ending, jam-packed schedules and extensive to-do lists all encompassing, work, home, family, community, and even ministry activities, vehemently crowding out time and space to connect with God on a deeper and personal level.

Excessive work without rest is a dangerous formula that only results in spiritual, physical, and mental fatigue, eventually leading to burnout.

Statistics from the American Institute of Stress reveal that stress is at an all-time high and shows no sign of slowing down [2].

- 3 out of 4 doctors' visits are for stress-related ailments

- 24% of US employees work 6+ extra hours weekly without pay, causing Americans to lose at least $2,262 per year (enough to take a family of five on a 5-day trip to Disney)

- Stress related ailments cost the nation $300 Billion annually in medical bills and lost productivity

- 44% of Americans feel more stressed than they did 5 years ago

- 1 in 5 Americans experience extreme stress to include heart palpitations, shaking and depression

- Work related stress causes 10% of all strokes

- 40% of people that are overly stressed overeat or eat unhealthy food

- 44% lose sleep every night

We Need a Remedy

People everywhere are desperately seeking answers to surmount the mountainous terrains of stress that they are facing. Every temporary remedy under the sun, ranging from sleep aids to prescription medications is proving to be inadequate in providing some form of permanent relief. We would do well to take a page from the book of Luke as Jesus loving and gently replies to his dear sister and friend Martha.

> *But Martha was distracted with much serving. And she went up to him and said, 'Lord, do you not care that my sister has left me to serve alone? Tell her then to help me,' but the Lord answered her, "Martha, Martha, you are anxious and troubled about many things, but one thing is necessary. Mary has chosen the good portion, which will not be taken away from her."*
>
> *Luke 10:40-42*

Mary was enjoying what I like to call a Sabbath moment. She purposefully took time to stop from all of her labor to sit down and be refilled and refreshed spiritually, physically, and mentally by the living waters found in Jesus' words. If we are not careful, much like Martha, we can become caught up by many of the daily activities of life and miss out on the goodness and blessings that God has for us when we rest in Him. Martha was greatly distracted by the activity of doing, creating an imbalance in her life. Like never before, Americans are being constantly bombarded with distractions from all sides: overbooked schedules, late night TV, social media platforms, video games, Reality TV shows, overspending, e-mails and cramming more work into longer working hours. As a wife, mom, veteran, business owner, minister, and community servant, this is something that I know all too well. While serving as a military Academic Instructor, I learned many valuable lessons about the delicate balance between work and rest.

My Experience

Being a military instructor is one of the most rewarding and fulfilling jobs, yet it is extremely mentally and physically demanding. Most of my days began at O'dark thirty, a military term, signifying very early hours of the morning well before daybreak. I would end many of my days late at night. For about 8 weeks straight, my team performed at highly demanding levels encompassing fitness, academic instruction, training, and team building and after eight weeks, we would have a two-week break in between each academic class. My weekends were filled with taking care of home and serving in ministry.

During the two-week breaks in between each class, my Commandant and senior leadership always gave specific orders, "you will do no work during your break." This time was committed to fun team building activities, light prep work for the next class and relaxation. By the time the next class came in, we were fully recharged and ready to re-engage with renewed levels of energy, enthusiasm, and focus. In a sense, the Sabbath has the same concept, work hard for six days and reserve one day for rest. I am blessed to live in an area that has a large Jewish community. One of the things I admire most about their culture is their honor and reverence in observing the Sabbath. On any given Friday afternoon, the city of Lakewood, New Jersey is all abuzz, as families prepare for the Sabbath, which begins early Friday evening and ends on Saturday evening.

On Friday evenings, the city is peacefully quiet. Stores and businesses are closed and families walk together to local synagogues for worship. On Saturday mornings, the city is still very quiet, as men walk to synagogues for worship, draped in their beautifully colored prayer shawls, often reading scriptures and reciting prayers. On one Friday evening, I remember driving through a housing development and came across a beautiful sight.

As I drove, the Holy Spirit drew my attention to look at a house on my left-hand side. As I looked up, the house had large bay windows that were wide opened and next to the windows sat a group of older Jewish men at a dining room table, teaching middle-aged men, teenage, and small boys from the Torah. As I gazed upon these men, young, and old, I began to grasp the sacred meaning of the Sabbath and why everything in the city stopped. Like Mary, to rest from all of one's labor, to connect with God, family, community, and nature by intently listening to the holy scriptures, preparing one's spirit, soul and body to confidently meet the challenges of life.

How Did America Become So Busy?

Growing up, I remember a time when America did cease from all of its working. It was rare to see businesses open on Sunday. Sunday was a day reserved for attending church services, enjoying family dinners, spending quality time with family, neighbors, and friends and relaxing. Regrettably, we have moved away from this practice and unlike our Jewish brethren, I do not believe that our nation fully grasped the essence of the Sabbath and inadvertently neglected this precious gift.

In my travels across the world, I have witnessed the stark difference between other countries and American culture; they simply are not as busy as we are. In European countries, it is written in their laws that every working person must take at least 30 days of vacation annually and they never miss their afternoon siestas, which are about three hours long. During this mid-day break from the hustle and bustle of work and life, businesses shut down, and individuals enjoy a home cooked meal shared amongst family and friends. Meal time is often followed by a leisurely nap. A friend of mine recounted a trip that she and her husband took to Europe and expressed how appalled she was that they could not be served lunch during siesta time. The business owner politely told them that this was their special time and to come back later. Not happy with this answer, she tried to persuade the owner to prepare their lunch based on the fact that they were Americans visiting from out of town and were quite hungry. However, she received the same response, come back later after our siesta is finished.

It's Time to Make an Adjustment

The first question that I usually get when I tell people that I served in the Air Force is, did you fly airplanes? Always smiling, I answer, no, but I have worked with some of the most outstanding flying units around the world. The closest that I've ever come to flying was during an informal training session on a C-5 flight simulator. The C-5, also known as the Galaxy because of its massive size, is one of the Air Force's largest transport aircrafts used to carry supplies, military personnel and equipment in support of global operations. If you've never been in a flight simulator, it's identical to being in the actual cockpit of a real airplane. Flight simulators create life-like scenarios in preparation of flying real aircraft in any and all conditions.

As I sat in the pilot's seat, I thought about how realistic the flight instruments and runway looked. I held the yoke and followed the instructions of the trained pilot who was with me. As the expert, he guided me with a confident and calming voice during the entire flight. When I got off course, he showed me how to make minor adjustments to navigate back on course. In much the same way, God is your pilot, and He wants to show you how to get back on course concerning the principles that govern spiritual, physical and mental rest. When we listen to His voice and take the necessary steps to follow His plan, we'll end up in the destination that He has already prepared for us.

> *The Lord is my Shepherd [to feed, guide, and shield me],*
> *I shall not lack. He makes me lie down in [fresh, tender]*
> *green pastures; He leads me beside the still and restful*
> *waters. He refreshes and restores my life (myself); He*
> *leads me in the paths of righteousness [uprightness and*

right standing with Him—not for my earning it, but] for His name's sake.

Psalms 23: 1-3

The Concepts of Rhythm and Time

The book of Genesis narrates how God created man from the dust of the earth. Because we were originally formed from the ground, we were designed to move naturally with the rhythm of the earth. There were no time constructs, regulating the day on a 24-hour system, only evening and morning. Ah, can you imagine a world with no schedules or constraints, just the evening and the morning! As the sun rose to meet the day, so did we, and when the sun descended for the evening, we retired, resting until the next day. Times certainly have changed. Our innate physical rhythm has been overridden by the erratic rhythm of American culture. The inception of night shifts, mid-day shifts, weekend shifts, and 24/7 operations have created negative rhythms and unpredictable patterns that have caused us to veer extremely off God's original course concerning rest. Rest is one of the most quintessential cornerstones of health, yet it receives little to no attention. Rest encompasses adequate sleep and taking the time to stop all forms of work.

What Happens to the Body During Sleep?

While we are sleeping, the body undergoes a natural healing process, recovering from the wear and tear the body experiences throughout the day. During this time of healing, blood cells, heart vessels, muscle tissues, joints, and ligaments are repaired. Hormones and blood sugar levels are properly regulated and the immune system and brain functions are strengthened. If an individual continues to follow erratic patterns and schedules, and does not provide the body with enough sleep, the following illnesses and problems can occur:

• Stroke

• Diabetes

- Obesity

- Irritability

- Heart disease

- Mood swings

- Kidney disease

- Immune deficiency

- Attention disorders

- Suicidal tendencies

- High blood pressure

- Psychological impairment

- Poor decision making ability

- Inability to control negative emotions and behavior

- Prone to having more accidents on the job and while driving

America is a Sleep Deprived and Overworked Nation

The National Sleep Foundation (NSF) discovered that millions of people are simply not getting enough sleep and many are suffering due to lack of sleep. Surveys conducted by the NSF (1999-2004) reveal that at least 40 million Americans suffer from over 70 different sleep disorders and 60 percent of adult's report having sleep problems a few nights a week or more. Most of those with these problems go undiagnosed and untreated [3]. More than 40 percent of adults experience daytime sleepiness severe enough to interfere with their daily activities at least a few days each month, with 20 percent reporting problem sleeping a few days a week or more [4]. Not only are adults being impacted by lack of sleep, 69 percent of children experience one or more sleep problems a few nights or more during a week [5]. These statistics present compelling evidence revealing that the direction we are headed in is not working. In order to bring your personal world into balance and alignment, proactive measures are necessary to guard the gift of rest.

It is vain for you to rise up early, to take rest late, to eat
the bread of toil, for so He gives unto his beloved sleep.
Psalms 127:2

How Much Sleep Do You Really Need?

The amount of sleep that each individual needs varies and is based on factors such as your age, exercise regiment, routines, and schedules, lifestyle, eating, and drinking habits. To operate at optimal levels, most health authority's state 8 hours of sleep is adequate for every 24-hour period [6]. Earlier, I mentioned the concept of learning how to listen to your body. If you are not feeling rested, ask yourself the following questions:

- At what time do I feel most fatigued?

- At what time do I feel most alert?

- How long does the fatigue or tiredness last?

- Do I fall asleep frequently at work or during routine activities?

- At what time do I go to bed every night?

- How do I feel upon rising?

These basic questions will help you to assess how much rest your body needs on a daily basis. Listening to your body is vital to determining whether or not you are meeting your sleeping needs. Once you determine how much you need, commit to make sleep a priority in your life, as well as protect your times of sleep. As you do, your body will begin to follow its innate rhythm for natural sleeping patterns. The results will yield an overall improvement in your health.

> *Sleep is that golden chain that ties health and our*
> *bodies together.*
>
> *Thomas Dekker*

The Intent of Remembering the Sabbath

The underpinning principles governing the Sabbath are connection with God, family, and rest. We live in an age filled with countless spiritual and natural influences that seem to magnetically pull us in so many directions. This disconnect leaves us severely deficient spiritually, mentally, and physically. The ideology of the Sabbath grants us permission to stop from all of our activities and allows us to capture the simplicity of purely being in the moment. For a brief time, we have God's sovereign permission to *not* check e-mails, run errands, answer phone calls, complete to-do lists or coordinate schedules. The gift of the Sabbath genuinely frees us from the busyness of our all-too-busy culture to provide rest for the body, soul and spirit.

The wonderful freedom that exists within the Sabbath has always been afforded to us, but we must choose to use this key wisely. When we intentionally rest from all of our labor, our awareness of God, family, friends, neighbors, and creation is heightened, enabling us to return back to our weekly activities with increased levels of energy, renewed enthusiasm, and fresh perspectives. The bible promises that when we delight in the Lord and follow the principles outlined for His people, we will experience greater blessings physically, mentally, and spiritually. Our heavenly Father gave us this commandment, not to keep us in bondage to the law, but as a way to experience the liberty, serenity, and rest that come as a result of embracing the true essence of the Sabbath.

> *If you turn away your foot from [traveling unduly on] the*
> *Sabbath, from doing your own pleasure on My holy day,*
> *and call the Sabbath a [spiritual] delight, the holy day*

of the Lord honorable, and honor Him and it, not going your own way or seeking or finding your own pleasure or speaking with your own [idle] words, Then will you delight yourself in the Lord, and I will make you to ride on the high places of the earth, and I will feed you with the heritage [promised for you] of Jacob your father; for the mouth of the Lord has spoken it.

Isaiah 58:13-14

Key # 6 - Remember the Sabbath...Rest for the
Spirit, Soul and Body

Healthy Ways to Rock Your World Naturally with the Sabbath

- Incorporate Sabbath moments into your life every week. Start off by looking at your schedule and determine what day of the week works best to rest from any and all working activities. This can be for a 24-hour period or whatever timeframe you chose that will work best for you. Commit to not allow anyone or anything to interfere with your time.

- Consider eliminating all electronic communications to include cell phones, ipads, TV's, computers and not wearing a watch during your chosen time of rest. To resist the temptation of engaging with your digital devices, silence or mute the ringers and keep them in a different room.

- Prepare a special meal and invite family, friends, and neighbors over. Make it a festive time by lighting candles and putting flowers on the dinner table. Before dinner, have each of your guests' share something that they are thankful or grateful for that God did for them during the week. After dinner, include a fun and relaxing activity like playing a board game.

- Include your children in your Sabbath moment. At some point during your time, read scriptures such as Psalms 127:3-5, Numbers 6:24-26 or Jeremiah 29:11 and pray a special blessing over your children to let them know how much God loves them, as well as how much you love and appreciate them.

- Take time to reconnect with God through prayer, meditation, scripture reading, and bible study or by journaling your thoughts about your Sabbath moment.

- Take an extra-long nap or candlelit bath to give your body the much-needed rest that it deserves.

- Refresh your body and mind by getting out into nature. Take a walk along a nature trail or visit your local park or beach to connect with God and His creation.

- Attend a bible-believing church regularly. Be prayerful about what day you choose as your main day of worship and commit to genuinely give your time and service to God.

- Make sleep a priority in your life. Assess how much sleep you really need. Experiment by taking 1-2 days during the week to not set your alarm clock. Allow your body to wake up naturally on its own to see how rested you feel.

- Turn your bedroom into a peaceful haven. Designate where you sleep as a rest and relaxation zone, free from work, distractions, clutter, and busy tasks i.e. working on the computer, watching television or paying bills. Ensure that your room is warm, relaxing, and comfortable. Diffuse calming Essential Oils such as Lavender, Sandalwood, or Frankincense in the area 15 minutes before resting.

- Take lunch breaks and allowable breaks on your job. Do not work through lunch. Even if it is for only 30-minutes, consider this as your personal siesta. Enjoy a healthy meal, read a good book or magazine or do something that you enjoy that is not work-related.

- During your Sabbath moment, rest in the permission that God has given you to not check e-mails, answer phone calls, coordinate schedules, balance bank accounts or run errands. Simply rest and discover pure enjoyment in the moment.

- Reflect on the blessings in your life i.e. family, friends, community, health, life, church etc. and thank God for them in prayer.

Key # 7

Healthy Habits to Preserve
and Protect Planet Earth

[Preserve / to maintain (something)
in its original or existing state]

Then God said, "Let us make man in our image,
in our likeness, and let them rule over the fish of the
sea and the birds of the air, over the livestock,
over all the earth, and over all the creatures
that move along the ground."

Genesis 1:26

You alone are the LORD. You made the heavens, even the highest heavens, and all their starry host, the earth and all that is on it, the seas and all that is in them. You give life to everything, and the multitudes of heaven worship you.
Nehemiah 9:6

Chapter 9

Protecting and Preserving Planet Earth

P salms 104 is one of my favorite Psalms. It is a spiritual song believed to be penned by David, expressing the deep dependence that all of creation has for God. It also speaks of the great interdependence between humans, animals, earth, plant life and oceans. We are all divinely connected and cannot exist without one another.

> ¹I praise you, Lord God, with all my heart.
> You are glorious and majestic, dressed in royal robes
> ² and surrounded by light. You spread out the sky
> like a tent,
> ³ and you built your home over the mighty ocean.
> The clouds
> are your chariots with the wind as its wings.
> ⁴ The winds are your messengers, and flames of fire are
> your servants.

⁵ You built foundations for the earth, and it will never be shaken.

⁶ You covered the earth with the ocean that rose above the mountains.

⁷ Then your voice thundered! And the water flowed
⁸ down the mountains and through the valleys to the place you prepared.

⁹ Now you have set boundaries, so that the water will never flood the earth again.

¹⁰ You provide streams of water in the hills and valleys,
¹¹ so that the donkeys and other wild animals can satisfy their thirst.

¹² Birds build their nests nearby and sing in the trees.

¹³ From your home above you send rain on the hills and water the earth.

¹⁴ You let the earth produce grass for cattle, plants for our food,
¹⁵ wine to cheer us up, olive oil for our skin, and grain for our health.

¹⁶ Our Lord, your trees always have water, and so do the cedars you planted in Lebanon.

¹⁷ Birds nest in those trees, and storks make their home in the fir trees.

¹⁸ Wild goats find a home in tall mountains, and small animals hide between the rocks.

¹⁹ You created the moon to tell us the seasons. The sun knows when to set,
²⁰ and you made the darkness, so the animals in the forest could come out at night.

²¹ Lions roar as they hunt for the food you provide.

²² But when morning comes, they return to their dens,
²³ then we go out to work until the end of day.

²⁴ Our Lord, by your wisdom you made so many things; the whole earth is covered
with your living creatures.

²⁵ But what about the ocean so big and wide? It is alive with creatures, large, and small.

[26] And there are the ships, as well as Leviathan, that you
created to splash in the sea.
[27] All of these depend on you to provide them with food,
[28] and you feed each one with your own hand, until
they are full.
[29] But when you turn away, they are terrified; when you
end their life, they die and rot.
[30] You created all of them by your Spirit, and you give
new life to the earth.

Psalms 104:1-30

As commissioned stewards over the earth, whatever actions we
make upon creation, whether positive or negative, a chain of events will
follow. In Matthew 24, Jesus forewarns His disciples of signs that will
occur as the day of Christ's return draws near, one of them being
weather phenomena on astronomical levels, specifically earthquakes in
diverse places. Within the past decade, the prophecy that Jesus spoke of
is being fulfilled, as various countries around the globe are experiencing
devastating earthquakes, tsunamis, volcanic eruptions, and mud slides
of epic proportions. These are spiritual signs signifying Jesus' return. I
also believe that the earth is crying out due to our poor stewardship over
our planet.

*And you will hear of wars and rumors of wars. See that
you are not alarmed, for this must take place, but the end
is not yet. For nation will rise against nation, and
kingdom against kingdom, and there will be famines and
earthquakes in various places.*

Matthew 24:6-7

The earth is in a chaotic state and is crying out with global warming,
earthquakes, forest fires, glacial melting, unpredictable weather patterns,
floods, storms, and droughts. In our ignorance, we have disrupted our
union with the earth by wastefully depleting its resources, in an effort to
fulfill our insatiable desire to consume and obtain more. Overburdening
the earth with toxic landfills, polluting vast oceans, seas, and rivers,
partaking in unsustainable agricultural practices, and creating greenhouse

emissions in massive quantities, have all resulted in a dangerous and unstable breach within our ecosystem.

The Earth is Alive

When God created the earth, He formed it out of His very Spirit, making it a spiritual entity, in fact a living organism. Yes, the earth is alive and continually declares God's glory. This is proven extensively throughout the bible.

> *Praise him, all heaven and earth! Praise him, all the seas and everything in them!*
>
> *Psalms 69:34*

> *The heavens are telling the glory of God; they are a marvelous display of his craftsmanship. Day and night, they keep on telling about God. Without a sound or word, silent in the skies, their message reaches out to all of the world. The sun lives in the heavens where God placed it and moves out across the skies as radiant as a bridegroom going to his wedding, or as joyous as an athlete looking forward to a race! The sun crosses the heavens from end to end, and nothing can hide from its heat.*
>
> *Psalms 19:1-6*

> *Praise the Lord, O heavens! Praise him from the skies! Praise him, all his angels, all the armies of heaven. Praise him, sun and moon and all you twinkling stars. Praise him, skies above. Praise him, vapors high above the clouds. Let everything he has made give praise to him. For he issued his command, and they came into being; he established them forever and forever. His orders will never be revoked. And praise him down here on earth, you creatures of the ocean depths. Let fire and hail, snow, rain, wind, and weather all obey. Let the mountains and hills, the fruit trees and cedars, the wild animals and cattle,*

the snakes and birds, the kings and all the people with their rulers and their judges, young men and maidens, old men and children - all praise the Lord together. For he alone is worthy. His glory is far greater than all of earth and heaven.

Psalms 148:1-13

As the rain and snow come down from heaven and stay upon the ground to water the earth, and cause the grain to grow and to produce seed for the farmer and bread for the hungry, so also is my word. I send it out, and it always produces fruit. It shall accomplish all I want it to and prosper everywhere I send it. You will live in joy and peace. The mountains and hills, the trees of the field - all the world around you - will rejoice.

Isaiah 55:10-12

The land suffers for the sins of its people. The earth languishes, the crops wither, the skies refuse their rain. The land is defiled by crime; the people have twisted the laws of God and broken his everlasting commands.

Isaiah 24:4-5

The words rejoice, praise, telling, and languish all denote some form of action or energy being released by the earth in expression to God. We have not treated the earth as if it were a part of God's living creation. I often wonder how God must feel about what we have done to the earth. We have reached a pivotal point in time, where we can no longer use excuses for not being faithful stewards over the planet that God has given us to inhabit. Just as our negative actions have resulted in adverse environmental repercussions, the same spiritual law holds true when we carry out good deeds, for whatsoever a man sows that shall he also reap.

Stewardship Over the Earth

We must return back to the position of responsibility. Collectively, we can begin practicing corrective measures to counter our negative behaviors, resulting in the betterment of our planet now and for future generations. The charge given to Adam to care for the earth has never changed. The seventh and final key is environmentally related, yet it is associated with all of the other keys. The food that we eat, the water that we drink, the air that we breathe, the resources that we use all come from our beautiful planet. In this chapter, I'll show you just how easy it is to implement simple everyday lifestyle habits that contribute to protecting and preserving Planet Earth. We'll start off with something that we all do, shopping.

Printed vs. Electronic Receipts

All over America, I am witnessing more organizations making an effort to heighten environmental awareness in their employees and customers. Going green is making an indelible footprint. During a trip to Staples, the cashier offered me the option of having my receipt e-mailed or printed. I opted for the e-mail to save on ink and paper. If you really think about it, what do most people do with their receipts? They are crumpled up and thrown in the trash, tucked away in glove compartments, or stuffed into pockets and purses never to be seen again. Some individuals may save them for business or tax purposes, but for the most part, receipts become faded and nothing is ever done with them. In 2012, Celerant Technology Corporation published a report outlining the statistics associated with the environmental and monetary cost of using printed receipts [1].

- In the U.S. alone, retailers consume 640,000 tons of thermal receipt paper per year, requiring 9.6 million trees for their manufacture.

- It takes approximately 390 gallons of oil to produce a single ton of paper. At 640,000 tons of thermal receipt paper demanded per year, that's nearly 250 million gallons of oil, enough to produce almost 16 million gallons of gas.

- The amount of CO2 emitted by producing one ton of receipt paper is equivalent to the amount of exhaust a car emits while driving for an entire year.

- It takes more than 19,000 gallons of water to produce a single ton of paper. This equates to more than 1.2 billion gallons of water used during the receipt paper production process.

- Approximately 2,278 pounds of trash is produced while producing a single ton of receipt paper. This means nearly 1.5 billion pounds of trash are being fed into landfills at the hands of receipt paper manufacturing.

In addition to wasting millions of resources annually, the ink used to print these receipts has been shown to contain BPA or Bisphenol-A, putting workers and customers at risk. When eating out and paying for your meal, the cashier usually places the receipt in your hand. Touching the receipt leaves traces of BPA on your hand, which in turn touches the food that you consume, entering your bloodstream. As previously mentioned, studies have shown that BPA exposure is associated with a multitude of health problems including infertility, weight gain, behavioral changes, early-onset puberty, prostate, and mammary gland cancers, endocrine disruption, cardiovascular effects and diabetes [2]. The health risks associated with printed receipts can be offset by simply going digital. The next time you're out shopping, ask about getting an electronic receipt e-mailed to you versus having one printed. If the store doesn't have this option, ask the store manager to consider implementing digital receipts at their place of business.

Reusable Bags vs. Paper and Plastic Bags

After shopping, we all need something to carry our merchandise home in. If you're at the grocery store, the cashier always asks what type of bags you prefer, paper, or plastic? Quite honestly, neither of these choices is better for the environment. In 2012, the United States generated 32 million tons of plastics waste from containers and packaging, and 7 million tons of non-durable plastic waste such as plates and cups. The combined total of nondurable disposables exceeded the 14 million tons of plastic durable goods, such as appliances. Only 9% was recovered for recycling [3]. That leaves a whopping 91% of plastic goods like non-biodegradable plastic bags that end up in landfills and littered across our country. This litter winds up in oceans, seas, streams, and lakes, often killing aquatic animals, plant life, and birds.

Manufacturing paper and plastic bags demands the use of a vast amount of resources. Plastic bags require 2.2 billion pounds of fossil fuel and 3.9 billion gallons of fresh water to produce the 100 billion plastic bags used annually in the United States [4]. As a result, a billion pounds of solid waste and 2.7 million tons of CO_2 are produced per year negatively contributing to global warming. Paper bags require the use of even more energy and water, creating more pollution. If that is not enough, 14 million trees are cut down annually to produce paper bags and US retailers spend $4 billion per year on disposable bags [5]. These distressing figures have motivated many countries and US cities to take action.

Ditching the Plastic Bag

In 2002, the Republic of Ireland became the first country to implement a plastic bag fee, also known as PlasTax [6]. The purpose of the PlasTax is to get consumers to change their behavior by not using plastic bags. If consumers use plastic bags at checkout they are required to pay a .15 cents fee for every used plastic bag. The results?

- Litter has been reduced dramatically

- Plastic bag consumption dropped by 94% from 1.2 billion to 230 million per year

- 18,000 liters of oil have been saved due to reduced production of bags

- Reusable shopping bags are taking the place of paper and plastic disposable bags

- Businesses are coming up with more eco-friendly choices for reusable bags rather than manufacturing paper or plastic bags

Because Ireland experienced such great success, other countries including Australia and South Africa have also imposed a plastic bag tax and are achieving the same results [7]. In like fashion, cities around the United States are embracing this green-minded movement by implementing legislative law to ban plastic bag use. To find out what cities in your state are active participants, you can use the Google search engine and type the words reuseit and Tools to Influence Policy. Once you are at the reuseit web site, click on the section that says Find Existing Single-Use Bag Legislation Near You. Just imagine the benefits our nation could experience over the next 5 to 10 years and beyond, if each household in America adopts the habit of using reusable bags. We would save on resources, protect the planet, cut down on wasteful spending, reduce the impact of global warming and inspire creative business ideas for more eco-friendly products.

Food Miles and Our Health

Have you ever taken the time to think about just how far your food has to travel before being delivered to grocery stores and eventually onto your plate? We are blessed to live in a nation that enjoys an endless list of diverse foods, drinks, and spices from around the world: oil from Italy, bell peppers from the Netherlands, rice from Thailand, grass-fed butter from New Zealand, bananas from Ecuador, meats from Australia, and coffee from Columbia.

Food is transported seamlessly and rapidly via the global highway by thousands of airplanes, ships, trains, boats, and trucks. This is known as food miles, or the distance food is transported from the time of its production until it reaches the consumer [8]. When broken down, this equates to the use of millions of gallons of fuel, packaging, storage space, pesticides, and processing. On average, produce arriving at major supermarkets is transported 1,500 miles or more [9]. Large companies and private sectors boast about the economic advantages of moving food globally, however, the environmental ramifications must be taken into account. Excluding dangerous gas emissions that come from food processing and production, transporting, disposing, and growing food within the US food supply chain, accounts for 13% of greenhouse gas emissions, contributing to climate change [10]. Climate change is the change in global or regional climate patterns and is attributed largely to increased levels of atmospheric carbon dioxide by the use of fossil fuels [11]. Climate change compromises our environmental resources and attributes to a decrease in safe drinking water, reduction in clean air quality and contaminates our healthy food supply and adversely affects our health.

The World Health Organization (WHO) estimates that the direct damage cost to health, excluding costs in health-determining sectors such as agriculture and water and sanitation, will be between $2-4 billion annually by 2030. Between 2030-2050, climate change will attribute to approximately 250,000 additional deaths per year, resulting from various diseases, to include asthma [12]. Organizations around the world such as WHO, are standing up and encouraging individuals to practice responsible and sustainable measures that preserve environmental health. We must also mobilize and become actively engaged by taking a proactive stance concerning where we purchase our food. We can all do our part by growing our own food or by purchasing the majority of our food locally.

The Benefits of Growing Your Own Food

Growing up, one of my most fond memories was helping my mother to plant our organic vegetable garden. My siblings and I helped mom plant all kinds of seeds: tomatoes, squash, lettuce, eggplant, corn, potatoes, peas, and carrots. My mother was careful to watch over the garden, teaching us how to pull up any weeds and remove any rocks that would choke out our harvest. She passed on to us, what she had learned from her parents and grandparents. Planting our organic garden did take some effort and it was more than worth it.

It was always exciting to watch the seeds blossom and grow. There was something very special about enjoying fresh vegetables from our family garden and having the food served right onto our plates. It was rewarding because we all had a part in growing our own food, we used no harmful chemicals or pesticides, and we knew exactly where it came from. Home grown food is extremely healthy and delicious, and we were also doing our part to sustain the earth. Another added benefit of growing our own food was that we saved money. Today, a pack of vegetable seeds such as tomatoes, squash, and eggplant or cucumbers costs roughly three dollars. Depending on what you purchase, this equates to the same cost as one pound of vegetables at the grocery store. If you're new to gardening, there are literally thousands of books and websites on the subject that will teach you how to grow your own food outdoors and indoors. If you're not ready to take the plunge to grow your own food, then the next best option is to buy local.

Why it Pays to Buy Your Food Locally

I am a regular shopper at my favorite local farmer's market. The particular market that I frequent offers excellent discounts on farm fresh organic cage free eggs, raw nuts, herbal teas, wild caught fish, unrefined oils, raw organic honey, nut milks, legumes, grains, fruits, and vegetables. Many local farmer's markets offer organic and non-GMO selections for even healthier food choices. Local farmers work diligently to produce food that is flavorful, rather than focusing on growing food that is rugged enough to transport thousands of miles around the world. When you ask most people why they shop at a farmer's market, it is because they believe that the quality and freshness of the food is better and they are also reassured that the food they are eating is produced by a local farmer and not grown in   a laboratory. Generally, local farmers transport food to markets that are within a 200-mile radius [13]. When you support your local farmer's market, not only are you doing something good for the earth, you are also helping to direct consumer spending towards the creation of new jobs and increase incomes in your community. Growing your own food or buying locally is a win-win situation on all fronts.

Mindless Consumption

America has become a nation that is plagued with overconsumption. Not more than a few decades ago, families prided themselves on knowing how to stretch a dollar to make ends meet, as well as using the resources they had on hand to create more of something. Growing up in a family of six, I experienced this first-hand. My parents always came up with creative ways to take care of the family. My siblings and I were thankful for what we had and we never seemed to lack anything. The opposite holds true today. Instead of being content, individuals are compelled to go out and purchase more of something. If you take an inventory of the average home, you will find closets and cabinets brimming and cluttered with things: clothes, shoes, papers, plastic containers, magazines, toys, supplies, digital devices, cleaning products etc., most of which may never be used or end up being tossed out, and eventually hauled off to a landfill.

We have removed ourselves from exercising mindful consumption to mindless consumption.

We purchase and accumulate things without giving thoughtfulness as to why we are making purchases. It is highly beneficial to incorporate what I like to call reflective moments into our shopping experiences prior to making purchases. Reflective moments are simple questions designed to heighten our awareness about responsible stewardship. Take time to reflect and consider the following: Do I really need this or do I already have something that I can use to fill the need? Am I being a good and faithful steward with my finances? How will my purchase impact the environment? Understand that I am not saying that we should not enjoy things, God has given us all things in life to enjoy; however, our overindulgence of consuming things mindlessly has become detrimental to the planet. It is imperative to consciously direct our thoughts towards taking care of the earth that God has blessed us with.

Then God said, "let us make human beings in our image, to be like us. They will reign over the fish in the sea, the birds in the sky, the livestock, all the wild animals on the earth, and the small animals that scurry along the ground." So God created human beings in his own image. In the image of God He created them, male and female He created them. Then God blessed them and said, "Be fruitful and multiply. Fill the earth and govern it. Reign over the fish in the sea, the birds in the sky, and all the animals that scurry along the ground."

Genesis 1:26-30

Choose Whole Food Over Packaged, Boxed, Canned, or Bottled Food

Earlier, I discussed the benefits of growing your own food or buying it from your local farmer's market. When you choose to purchase unpackaged whole foods instead of buying food in packages, boxes, cans, or bottles you are protecting the environment by eliminating the outer packing. Because recycling is not routinely practiced, outer packing ends up in landfills further polluting the earth. In 2012, Americans generated about 251 million tons of trash and recycled and composted almost 87 million tons of this material, equivalent to a 34.5% recycling rate, leaving 65.5% of items in landfills un-recycled [14].

Our rate of consumption is exceeding our ability to recycle every year. Recycling helps to reduce waste, but the process releases a large quantity of greenhouse emissions into the environment. Millions of the items that remain in landfills decompose and leak into the earth, polluting the soil and groundwater. Rather than contributing to the problem, the best remedy is to purchase whole food without the packaging. Unpackaged, living whole food provides nourishment to the body that processed packaged food cannot. If you take it one step further, you can bring along reusable containers or smaller reusable bags to carry your produce in and bigger reusable bags to wrap your food in. Purchasing unpackaged food is just one of the many thousands of ways that you can begin reducing excessive waste. Embracing healthier lifestyle habits to preserve and protect the earth, can result in reaping huge dividends financially and environmentally, and can also include common items we all use every day such as paper towels and napkins.

Paper Towels & Paper Napkins Are Way Overrated!

Growing up, I never remember using paper towels or paper napkins except on a few rare occasions. We always had cloth napkins or just washed our hands if things got too messy. Nowadays, grocery store shelves are lined with various brands of paper towels and napkins claiming to have the quickest and best absorption rates. Millions of individuals are spending their hard-earned dollars on something that is wasted and tossed into the trash, with paper taking up as much as 50% of all landfill space [15].

The National Resources Defense Council recorded that, forests in America and Canada are being cut down at an incredible rate every year, disrupting the ecosystem, and destroying the habitation for countless species [16]. Due to the ongoing demand from tissue companies, logging claims half a million acres of Ontario and Alberta's boreal forest annually, a primeval expanse of pine, spruce, fir, and poplar trees that nourishes caribou, lynx, bear, wolves, and scores of songbirds. The native forests of the southeastern United States are also vanishing in massive numbers. These fragile ecosystems support dense stands of oak, hickory, black gum and red maple, and provide a haven for deer, fox, and more than 230 fish species. When forests are destroyed, it takes several decades for these woodlands to repopulate and grow. In reality, the Dr. Seuss movie, *The Lorax,* is not far off from being fulfilled.

How Much Are Paper Products Costing Us?

Although paper napkins and paper towels only serve as a small sector of the paper manufacturing industry, we must candidly ask, is what we are doing to creation for the sake of having paper goods worth it? To shed further light on this issue, here are some statistics on paper towels and what they are actually costing our nation [17, 18].

- To make one ton of paper towels 17 trees and 20,000 gallons of water are polluted

- Every day, over 3,000 tons of paper towel waste is produced in the U.S. alone

- Decomposing paper towels produces methane gas, a leading cause of global warming

- In the U.S., we currently use more than 13 billion pounds of paper towels each year and that number is growing steadily. This equates to more than 3,000 tons of paper towel waste in the U.S. alone

- Globally, discarded paper towels result in 254 million tons of trash every year

- As many as 51,000 trees per day are required to replace the number of paper towels that are discarded every day

- If every household in the U.S. used just one less 70-sheet roll of paper towels, that would save 544,000 trees each year

- If every household in the U.S. used three less rolls per year, it would save 120,000 tons of waste and $4.1 million in landfill dumping fees

A Call to Responsible Stewardship

A call to responsible stewardship not only encompasses monetary values, but it also involves how we take care of the earth. The earth is a priceless treasure, God's spiritual incubator that provides us with food, protection, shelter, and clothing. While it is true that we have made mistakes in the past, we can move forward with renewed mindsets and responsible approaches concerning our relationship with the earth and how our actions affect it.

God took the time to dedicate six whole days to prepare and create everything in the earth just for us and He wants us to appreciate and enjoy its countless blessings by respecting and cherishing the gift. The idea of protecting and preserving the earth may be a new concept for many, yet this has always been God's way. He never changes and is the same yesterday, today, and forever. We must diligently work towards restoring the sacred relationship between earth and humanity and return back to the place of responsibility that glorifies God, honors the earth and brings healing to our land. May we accept this call and commit to embrace His ways until His triumphant return.

> *...the land is mine and you reside in my land as foreigners and strangers. Throughout the land that you hold as a possession, you must provide for the redemption of the land.*
>
> *Leviticus 25:23-24*

> *Then if my people who are called by my name will humble themselves and pray and seek my face and turn from their wicked ways, I will hear from heaven and will forgive their sins and restore their land.*
>
> *2 Chronicles 7:14*

Key # 7 - Healthy Habits to Preserve Planet Earth

Healthy Ways to Rock Your World Naturally
by Protecting & Preserving Planet Earth

- Use Reusable bags. Shop at stores that promote the use of reusable bags. Whole Foods Market offers a .10 cent discount for each bag you use. Over the course of one year, those dimes can equate to savings that can be used for a rainy day.

- Be proactive and be a part of the anti-plastic bag movement. If the businesses you frequent don't offer incentives for using recyclable bags, talk to the store manager about implementing a program. When you speak to him/her, focus on the benefits of saving money for their company, as well as protecting and preserving the environment.

- Get involved! Find out what cities in your state are active participants in the anti-plastic bag movement by visiting www.reusit.com. Click on Tools to Influence Policy and then click on Find Existing Single-Use Bag Legislation Near You.

- Consider decreasing your paper towel or paper napkin usage and rely more on cloth hand towels. At home, keep one roll of paper towels or one package of napkins in an inconspicuous place and only use them in case of emergency spills or cleanups.

- Opt for using e-receipts versus printed receipts. The next time you're at the checkout counter, ask to have your receipt e-mailed or texted to you. If you're concerned about tracking your expenses and feel that you need paper, keep a small notepad and pen handy to help you keep track. Or even better, solely rely on electronic banking to eliminate all paper.

- Grow your own food. Take up organic gardening or support your local community garden. If you don't have an organic community garden, think about partnering with your church, synagogue or local organization to start one.

- Buy local. Find out where the local farmers markets are in your city or town and plan a trip by visiting www.localharvest.org. You'll discover that not only will you save money, but you'll also be supporting local farmers and preserving the earth.

- Not only is BPA used in thermal paper receipts, it is also found in other forms of printed media such as tickets, newspapers, and magazines. Opt to use the electronic version when purchasing any of these items.

- Skip the landfills and recycle old furniture, toys, clothes, household items and electronics. Use community resources to donate items you no longer want. A few good places to donate reusable goods are to your local church, parish, friends, neighbors, veteran's organizations, www.freecycle. com, www.craigslist.com, www.habitatforhumanity.org, www.donationtown.org and www.salvationarmy.org.

- Choose whole food without the packaging over boxed, packaged, canned, or bottled food. Not only is whole food healthier, you'll be doing your part to help remedy the ever-growing burden of landfills.

- Use reflective moments to help you avoid compulsive spending. Ask yourself the following questions: Do I really need this or do I already have something that will fill this need? Am I being a good and faithful steward with my finances and over the earth? How will my purchase impact the earth?

- Visit www.1800recycling.com and www.reuseit.com to discover the thousands of ways you can help to reduce waste on the planet. Practice being green-minded while on the go and download the 1.800.Recycling app on your smartphone.

The Health Revolution is Now

*[Revolution / a forcible overthrow of a government
or social order in favor of a new system]*

*Do not be conformed to this world (this age),
[fashioned after and adapted to its external,
superficial customs and systems], but be transformed
(changed) by the [entire] renewal of your mind
[by its new ideals and its new attitude], so that you may
prove [for yourselves] what is the good and
acceptable and perfect will of God, the thing which
is good and acceptable and perfect [in His sight for you].*

Romans 12:2

We use God's mighty weapons, not worldly weapons, to knock down the strongholds of human reasoning and to destroy false arguments.
2 Corinthians 10:4

Chapter 10

Will You Join the Health Revolution?

This book was written out of my deep love and desire to share the message of health as revealed within the bible. As we witness the plight of our crumbling healthcare system, each passing day reveals that it is becoming more and more of an enigma. Rather than providing effective long-term healing solutions, it has become a system filled with convoluted medical terminology, dangerous pharmaceuticals and business model approaches that negate the health of the whole person. While all of the blame cannot be shifted onto a faulty system, we must take personal responsibility concerning our actions regarding our health. God's approach to health has always been holistic embodying spirit, soul and body. Rather than embracing His original health plan, we have replaced it with ineffective practices that the body was never fashioned to withstand.

*Now may the God of peace make you holy in every way,
and may your whole spirit and soul and body be kept
blameless until our Lord Jesus Christ comes again.*
                                        I Thessalonians 5:23

The spirit, soul, and body each have a different function, yet they cannot be approached separately because they were designed to operate synergistically. For what influences the spirit, influences the soul and what influences the soul influences the body. This is witnessed when a person dies. When a person's spirit leaves their physical body, the whole body ceases to function. Created in the likeness and image of our Creator, manifested as Father, Son, and Holy Spirit, they are separate, but one. During Jesus' earthly ministry, He said, I can do nothing by myself, my Father and I are one. The Holy Spirit is the very personality of God, living and dwelling within us. These illustrations are presented to emphasize the reality that our spirituality should never be disconnected from our physiology. Our physical health and well-being cannot be successfully approached with systems outside of God's original design.

*We are not human beings having a spiritual experience.
We are spiritual beings having a human experience.*
                                        Pierre Teilhard de Chardin

The consequences of not addressing our health needs in alignment to God's holistic system have created dysfunction in grave proportions spiritually, physically, emotionally, socially, environmentally, and financially. It is time to cast off and let go of systems that were never meant for us regarding our health. As God has revealed through the scriptures in Leviticus 17:11, our physical health and healing begins and ends with our blood cells. We must diligently strive to keep our blood cells healthy, strong, and full of energy by embracing and living out the seven biblical keys. When God formed Adam from the dust, He breathed the breath of life, His very Spirit into him, and at the point of contact, blood began to flow throughout Adam's body. The very life of God flowed through Adam's veins in the form of blood. The blood is not only a physical liquid substance; its' very essence is spiritual because it came from God himself who is Spirit.

200

As spiritual beings, living in a physical body, we must remain within the boundaries of spiritual laws designed by God to protect and maintain our health. Now more than ever before, we must return to our Father's ways, ways that when followed, will lead us down the pathway of health that God has always reserved for us from the beginning of time. None of us knows the day nor the hour when we will go home to be with the Lord or when Jesus Christ will return for His church, but while we are here on earth, His will is that we live our days out fully in health and wholeness in spirit, soul and body.

There is a health revolution sweeping across America. Men, women, and children are no longer putting their faith in faulty systems and ineffective methods, but are seeking alternative answers to live healthier. Who better to obtain those answers from than from the Creator who fashioned us with His own two hands?

It is time to launch a God-inspired revolution in favor of a new system that is not really new, but has always belonged to us, the God-care system.

No longer conforming to the systems of this world, but wholly living God-centered biblical principles that result in transformation in spirit, soul and body. I invite you to adopt this new approach to health. To do so will involve your willingness to let go of the old mindsets and ineffective methods in favor of God's system to prove what is good, acceptable, and His perfect will towards living a healthy life.

The seven divine keys to unlock extraordinary health are far from complicated; in fact they are quite simple. The scriptures remind us that God has chosen the simple things to confound the wise, so it is not necessary to over think the principles. Because people are so accustomed to practicing health treatments that have proven to be altogether too complex, they are continually amazed at how simple and effective it is to implement the seven keys. When practiced consistently, all of the keys operate harmoniously to keep the blood cells functioning at optimal levels of health.

- Key # 1 - Fresh Air through Exercise & Healthy Lifestyle Habits

- Key # 2 - Love, Protect & Nurture Your Skin

- Key # 3 - Eat Clean Organic Non-GMO Food & Eliminate All Processed Food

- Key # 4 - Drink Clean Filtered Water

- Key # 5 - Incorporate Essential Oils Into Your World

- Key #6 - Remember the Sabbath...Rest for the Body, Soul & Spirit

- Key #7 - Healthy Habits to Protect & Preserve Planet Earth

My prayer for the church is that we will rise up, not to just become a part of the revolution, but that we take a leading role in the health revolution. God needs his church healthy, equipped, and ready to stand strong for this end time generation. As God's army, we cannot fight the good fight of faith or be effective for the Kingdom of God if we are not physically or spiritually fit. May these seven keys serve you well on your journey to health and wholeness. Divine healing is part of your God-given birthright and now is time for you to possess the promise. The health revolution is here. The health revolution is now. Will you join the revolution?

ROCK YOUR WORLD NATURALLY

I pray that you were blessed by this book.

Visit my web site at www.rockyourworldnaturally.com and click on the book tab. There you'll find a resource link containing resources to help you on your wellness journey.

What did you find most helpful about this book?

For the next 28-days, choose at least 7 areas, one key from each chapter that you will begin incorporating into your daily lifestyle and let me know how you're doing by e-mailing me at rockyourworldnaturally@gmail.com.

Stay Connected:

Twitter @RockYourWorld28

Facebook/RockYourWorldNaturally

Intsagram/RockYourWorldNaturally

Beloved, I pray that you may prosper in every way and [that your body] may keep well, even as [I know] your soul keeps well.

3 John 2

References

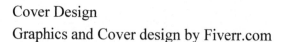

Cover Design

Graphics and Cover design by Fiverr.com

Preface

1. Bipartisan Policy Center, September 2012. "What is Driving U.S. Health Care Spending?"

2. Pricewaterhouse Coopers Health Research Institute, April 2008. "The Price of Excess: Identifying Waste in Healthcare Spending."

3. Dartmouth Institute for Health Policy and Clinical Practice. "The State of the Nation's," Spring 2007.

4. Common Wealth Fund, U.S. Health System Ranks Last Among Eleven Countries Based on Measures of Access, Equity, Quality, Efficiency, and Healthy Lives

    http://www.commonwealthfund.org/~/media/files/news/news-releases/2014/mirror-mirror-release-final-6_13_14.pdf

Chapter 1 – In the Beginning

1. Blood: The River of life, Herald Tribune http://www.heraldtribune.com/article/20110906/ARTICLE/110909759

2. http://en.wikipedia.org/wiki/Blood

3. Health Hazards of Chemicals http://web.princeton.edu/
sites/ehs/labsafetymanual/sec5.htm#routes

4. Industrial Revolution Major Problems in Urban History
Documents and Essays, The City in American History,
Arthur M. Schlesinger pgs 1-12, 1994

Chapter 2 – Fresh Air
Inhale definition –
https://www.google.com/
search?q=revolution+definition&rlz=1C1SNNT_
enUS447&oq=revolution+definition&aqs=
chrome.0.0l6.3687j1j4&sourceid=chrome&es_sm=93&ie=UTF-
8#q=inhale+definition
  1. National Heart, Lung, and Blood Institute. What Happens
When You Breathe? http://www.nhlbi.nih.gov/health/
health-topics/topics/hlw/whathappens

     What is Respiratory Failure? http://www.nhlbi.nih.gov/
health/health-topics/topics/rf

  2. Medical Problems in High Mountain Environments: A
Handbook for Medical Officers,

     US Army -Research Institute of Environmental Medicine
Natick, Massachusetts 01760-5007

     Allen Cymerman, Ph.D. and Paul B. Rock, LTC, MC
February 1994

     http://archive.rubicon-foundation.org/xmlui/bitstream/
handle/123456789/7976/ADA278095.pdf?sequence=1

  3. Oxygen: Health Effects and Regulatory Limits Part
I: Physiological and Toxicological Effects of Oxygen
Deficiency and Enrichment Neil McManus, CIH, ROH,

CSP Northwest Occupational Health & Safety North Vancouver, British Columbia, Canada nwohs@mdi.ca www.nwohs.com

http://www.nwohs.com/Oxygen%20Regulatory%20 Limits%20I.pdf

4. Forest therapy' taking root: Researchers find that a simple stroll among trees has real benefits by Akaemi Nakmura http://www.japantimes.co.jp/news/2008/05/02/national/ forest-therapy-taking-root/#.VQl_dI7F8ig

5. Vitamin D Fact Sheet for Professionals http://ods.od.nih. gov/factsheets/VitaminD-HealthProfessional/

5. Morbidity is Related to a Green Living Environment, Maas, J., Verheij, R.A., Vries, S. de, Spreeuwenberg, P., Groenewegen, P.P., Schellevis, F.G. Morbi~i ;) related to a green living environment. Journal of Epidemiology & Community Health: 2009, 63(12), 96

6. Vitamin D Status: United States, 2001–2006 http://www. cdc.gov/nchs/data/databriefs/db59.htm, Anne C. Looker, Ph.D.; Clifford L. Johnson, M.P.H.; David A. Lacher, M.D.; Christine M. Pfeiffer, Ph.D.; Rosemary L. Schleicher, Ph.D.; and Christopher T. Sempos, Ph.D.

7. "The Nobel Prize in Physiology or Medicine 1931". *Nobelprize.org.* Nobel Media AB 2014. Web. 15 Mar 2015. http://www.nobelprize.org/nobel_prizes/ medicine/laureates/1931/

8. Medical Definition of ANAEROBIOSIS. : life in the absence of air or free oxygen.

http://www.merriam-webster.com/dictionary/anaerobiosis

9. http://www.nndb.com/people/682/000127301/ Ottoburg

10. http://www.epa.gov/region1/communities/indoorair.html

11. New York Times, September 29, 1997, "New Toxins Suspected as Cancer Rate Rises in Children"

12. National Report on human Exposure to Environmental Chemicals http://www.cdc.gov/exposurereport/

13. The toxic chemicals in household cleaners are three times more likely to cause cancer than air pollution http://www.epa.gov/iaq/

14. Indoor Air Facts No. 4 (revised) Sick Building Syndrome http://www.epa.gov/iaq/pdfs/sick_building_factsheet.pdf

15. The EPA has deemed poor indoor air quality as one of the top five health hazards of our time http://www.epa.gov/iaq/

16. Benefits of Improving Indoor Environmental Quality http://www.iaqscience.lbl.gov/benefits-summary.html

17. Asthma Prevalence in the US http://www.cdc.gov/asthma/asthmadata.htm

18. Illnesses associated with indoor toxins http://www.epa.gov/iaq/

19. Substance Control Act 1976 http://www.epa.gov/agriculture/lsca.html,

20. What is a Toxic Substance? http://www.epa.gov/pesticides/kids/hometour/toxic.htm

21. Too Fight to Fight Too Fat to Fight http://cdn.missionreadiness.org/MR_Too_Fat_to_Fight-1.pdf

22. Overweight and Obesity http://www.cdc.gov/obesity/data/facts.html

23. Lower Direct Medical Costs Associated with Physical Activity

    http://www.cdc.gov/media/pressrel/r2k1006a.htm

24. World Health Organization Future Use of Materials for Dental Restoration http://www.who.int/oral_health/publications/dental_material_2011.pdf

25. About Dental Amalgam Fillings http://www.fda.gov/MedicalDevices/ProductsandMedicalProcedures/DentalProducts/DentalAmalgam/ucm171094.htm

26. Holistic Dentistry http://en.wikipedia.org/wiki/Holistic_dentistry

Chapter 3 - Skin

Absorption definition - https://www.google.com/search?q=revolution+definition&rlz=1C1SNNT_enUS447&oq=revolution+definition&aqs=chrome.0.0l6.3687j1j4&sourceid=chrome&es_sm=93&ie=UTF-8#q=absorption+definition

1. Phlebotomy Essentials by Ruth E. McCall, Cathee M. Tankersley, page 70

2. Skin Problems & Treatments Health Center

   http://www.webmd.com/skin-problems-and-treatments/picture-of-the-skin

3. http://www.fda.gov

4. http://www.fda.gov

5. Agency for Toxic Substances and Disease Registry (ATSDR) - Dibutyl phthalate - http://www.atsdr.cdc.gov/substances/toxsubstance.asp?toxid=167

6. Report on Carcinogens, Thirteenth Edition National Toxicology Program, Department of Health and Human Services For - Formaldehyde CAS No. 50-00-0 Known to be a human carcinogen First listed in the Second Annual Report on Carcinogens (1981) http://ntp.niehs.nih.gov/ntp/roc/content/profiles/formaldehyde.pdf

7. Triclosan - http://www.cir-safety.org/sites/default/files/FR569.pdf

8. Butylparaben [CAS No. 94-26-8] Review of Toxicological Literature http://ntp.niehs.nih.gov/ntp/htdocs/chem_background/exsumpdf/butylparaben_508.pdf

9. Report on Carcinogens http://ntp.niehs.nih.gov/pubhealth/roc/index.html

10. Edward Scripture, The New Psychology (1897): The original 1872 experiment was cited in: Sedgwick, "On the Variation of Reflex Excitability in the Frog induced by changes of Temperature," Stud. Biol. Lab. Johns Hopkins University (1882): 385.

11. Autoimmune diseases http://www.niaid.nih.gov/topics/autoimmune/Pages/default.aspx

12. Common autoimmune disorders http://www.nlm.nih.gov/medlineplus/ency/article/000816.htm

Volume 10, Number 11—November 2004, THEME ISSUE IEID & ICWID 2004 International Conference on Women and Infectious Diseases (ICWID) National

Institute of Health – Auto Immune Diseases Coordination Committee, Autoimmune Diseases Research Plan

http://www.niaid.nih.gov/topics/autoimmune/documents/adccreport.pdf

13. Cosmetic expenses http://www.commerce.gov/

14. Natural Food Definition http://en.wikipedia.org/wiki/Natural_foods

15. Alan Reinstein and Trevor Schaefer Toxic Chemical Protection Act https://www.congress.gov/bill/114th-congress/senate-bill/725/actions

16. European Union Ban Animal Testing http://ec.europa.eu/growth/sectors/cosmetics/animal-testing/index_en.htm

Chapter 4 – Injection Tattoos
Injection definition –
https://www.google.com/search?q=revolution+definition&rlz=1C1SNNT_enUS447&oq=revolution+definition&aqs=chrome.0.0l6.3687j1j4&sourceid=chrome&es_sm=93&ie=UTF-8#q=injection+definition
1. Safe Injection Global Network: Advocacy booklet

http://www.who.int/injection_safety/sign/advocacy_booklet/en/

2. Tattoos Jamieson-Fausset-Brown Bible Commentary http://biblehub.com/commentaries/jfb//leviticus/19.htm

3. US National Library of Medicine National Institutes of Health, 2001; 5(1):27-34.

   Tattoos as risk factors for transfusion-transmitted diseases.

   http://www.ncbi.nlm.nih.gov/pubmed/11285156

4. Think Before You Ink: Are Tattoos Safe http://www.fda.gov/ForConsumers/ConsumerUpdates/ucm048919.htm

5. Maya Angelou http://en.wikipedia.org/wiki/Maya_Angelou

6. Mother Theresa http://en.wikipedia.org/wiki/Mother_Teresa#Commemoration

7. Botulinum toxin http://www.ncbi.nlm.nih.gov/pmc/articles/PMC2856357/

   Indian J Dermatol. 2010 Jan-Mar; 55(1): 8–14. doi:

8. FDA approves Botox Cosmetic to improve the appearance of crow's feet lines http://www.fda.gov/NewsEvents/Newsroom/PressAnnouncements/ucm367662.htm

9. Tests and Procedures: Botox Injections, The Mayo Clinic http://www.mayoclinic.org/tests-procedures/botox/basics/risks/prc-20009036

10. Children's Vaccine Quote http://www.cdc.gov/vaccines/schedules/downloads/child/0-18yrs-child-combined-schedule.pdf

11. Thimerosal in Vaccines http://www.fda.gov/BiologicsBloodVaccines/SafetyAvailability/VaccineSafety/UCM09622

12. Thimerosal in Vaccines http://www.fda.gov/
    biologicsbloodvaccines/safetyavailability/vaccinesafety/
    ucm096228.htm#t

13. Thimerosal in Vaccines Quote http://www.niaid.nih.gov/
    topics/vaccines/research/pages/vaccines.aspx

14. Methyl Mercury Side Effects http://www.epa.gov/mercury/
    effects.htm#meth

15. Centers for Disease Control, 2013 "Vaccine Excipient
    & Media Summary." http://www.cdc.gov/vaccines/pubs/
    pinkbook/downloads/appendices/B/excipient-table-2.pdf

16. National Vaccine Injury Compensation Program (VICP)
    Adjudication Categories by Vaccine for Claims Filed
    01/01/2006 through 12/31/2013 http://www.hrsa.gov/
    vaccinecompensation/statisticsreport.pdf

17. $3 Billion Payout http://www.cdc.gov/vaccinesafety/
    Activities/vaers.html Centers for Disease Control
    and Prevention - Vaccine Adverse Event Reporting
    System (VAERS)

18. Quote - Vaccine Effectiveness - How Well Does the Flu
    Vaccine Work? Centers for Disease Control and Prevention
    http://www.cdc.gov/flu/about/qa/vaccineeffect.htm

Dorland's Medical Dictionary for Health Consumers
    - Neurotoxins are substances that are poisonous or
    destructive to nerve tissue

19. Banned in Sweden, Norway, and Finland

    http://www.food.gov.uk/sites/default/files/multimedia/
    pdfs/publication/guidelinessotonsixcolours.pdf, http://
    www.telegraph.co.uk/news/health/news/3453522/

The-additives-which-could-be-banned.html, https://web. archive.org/web/20130909224854/http://www.cbc.ca/news/ background/foodsafety/additives.html

Chapter 5 - Ingestion
Ingestion Definition - www.merriam-webster.com/medical/ingestion

1. Food product definition http://www.thefreedictionary.com/ food+product

2. Nicholas Appert Issues the First Book on Modern Food Preservation Methods

   http://www.historyofinformation.com/expanded. php?id=2541

3. GIGO definition http://techterms.com/definition/gigo

4. Pesticides on Food http://www.panna.org/issues/ food-agriculture/pesticides-on-food

5. Chemical Trespass: Pesticides in Our Bodies and Corporate Accountability http://www.panna.org/sites/default/files/ ChemTresMain(screen).pdf

6. US Environmental Protection Agency Pesticide Industry Sales and Usage 2006-2007 Market Estimates

   http://www.epa.gov/opp00001/pestsales/07pestsales/ market_estimates2007.pdf

7. Organic food http://en.wikipedia.org/wiki/Organic_food

8. Health Risks of Pesticides in Food http://www.depts. washington.edu

9. Health Risks of Pesticides in Food http://www.depts. washington.edu

10. WHO GMO definition http://www.who.int/topics/ food_genetically_modified/en/

11. GMO Engineered Foods http://www.nlm.nih.gov/ medlineplus/ency/article/002432.htm

12. GMO's and Your Family http://www.nongmoproject.org/ learn-more/gmos-and-your-family/

13. Countries Growing GMO's http://www.gmo-compass. org/eng/agri_biotechnology/gmo_planting/142.countries_ growing_gmos.html

14. Vanishing Bees http://www.vanishingbees.com/

15. The Rise of the Super Weeds And What to Do About It http://www.ucsusa.org/food_and_agriculture/our-failing-food-system/industrial-agriculture/the-rise-of-superweeds.html

16. Impacts of genetically engineered crops on pesticide use in the U.S. – the first sixteen years http://www.enveurope. com/content/pdf/2190-4715-24-24.pdf

17. GMO Myths and Truths http://responsibletechnology.org/ GMO-Myths-and-Truths-edition2.pdf

18. Complete Genes May Pass from Food to Human Blood, Editor: Andrew Dewan, Yale School of Public Health, United States of America Received September 25, 2012; Accepted June 4, 2013; Published July 30, 2013 http://www.plosone.org/article/ fetchObject.action?uri=info:doi/10.1371/journal. pone.0069805&representation=PDF

GMOs linked to gluten disorders plaguing 18 million Americans - report

Published time: November 26, 2013 20:20 Edited time: November 28, 2013 14:20

http://rt.com/usa/gmo-gluten-sensitivity-trigger-343/

19. Republished study: long-term toxicity of a Roundup herbicide and a Roundup-tolerant genetically modified maize Séralini et al. Environmental Sciences Europe 2014, 26:14 http://www.enveurope.com/content/26/1/14http://www.enveurope.com/content/pdf/s12302-014-0014-5.pdf

20. Twenty-Six Countries Ban GMOs—Why Won't the US? Walden Bello and Foreign Policy In Focus on October 29, 2013 - 11:59 AM ET

    http://www.thenation.com/blog/176863/twenty-six-countries-ban-gmos-why-wont-us

21. It's Official, Russia Has Banned GMO Products. Commitment to Organic Food

    By Global Research News, Global Research, November 19, 2014

    http://www.globalresearch.ca/its-official-russia-has-banned-gmo-products-commitment-to-organic-food/5414961?print=1

22. Global Animal Partnershiphttp://www.globalanimalpartnership.org/

23. The 5-Step Program http://www.globalanimalpartnership.org/the-5-step-program/

24. Attitudes Toward the FDA's Plan on Genetically Engineering Fish, Americans in Near Unanimity in Their Disapproval of Genetically Engineered Fish and Meat in the Marketplace, Lake Research, September 20, 2010

25. Right to Know Act Bill S.809 https://www.govtrack.us/congress/bills/113/s809

26. Fast Food Nation: The Dark Side of the All-American Meal, by Eric Schlosser. Boston: Houghton Mifflin, 2001. ISBN: 039597 (p 3)

27. Estimates of Food Borne Illness in the US http://www.cdc.gov/foodborneburden/

28. Eat Right for Your Type: The Individualized Diet Solution to Staying Healthy, Living Longer & Achieving Your Ideal Weight, Peter J. D'Adamo with Catherine Whitney

Chapter 6 – Water

Water Definition – WikiPedia https://www.google.com/?gws_rd=ssl#q=water+definition
1. Water covers 70% of the earth's surface http://www.nasa.gov/missions/science/f_water.html

2. Body comprised of water https://water.usgs.gov/edu/propertyyou.html

3. Functions of water in the body http://www.mayoclinic.org/healthy-living/nutrition-and-healthy-eating/multimedia/functions-of-water-in-the-body/img-20005799

4. Statistics on not drinking water http://www.cdc.gov/pcd/issues/2013/12_0248.htm

5. Girls who don't drink water http://www.
    theatlantic.com/health/archive/2014/04/
    the-girl-who-wouldnt-drink-water/360342/

6. Your Body's Many Cries for Water: You're Not Sick;
    You're Thirsty, Don't Treat Thirst with Medication, F.
    Batmanghelidj, M.D.

7. American Heart Association Sugar
    Overload http://blog.heart.org/
    life-is-sweet-but-shouldnt-involve-this-much-sugar/

8. 10 Easy Paths to Self Destruction, Ohio State University
    Psychologist Brad Lander

9. Mayo Clinic sugar in the blood – blood cells http://www.
    mayoclinic.org/diseases-conditions/diabetes/expert-blog/
    high-blood-sugar/bgp-20056519

10. Adapted from 146 Reasons Why Sugar Is Ruining Your
    Health by Nancy Appleton, Ph.D.

11. WHO 2.6 Billion no water http://www.who.int/
    water_sanitation_health/mdg1/en/

12. Institute of Medicine http://www.iom.com

13. Symptoms of Dehydration in Adults http://www.
    emedicinehealth.com/dehydration_in_adults/page3_em.htm

14. 98.6 degree body temperature doi: 10.1128/mBio.00212-
    109 November 2010 mBio vol. 1 no. 5 e00212-10
    Mammalian Endothermy Optimally Restricts Fungi and
    Metabolic Costs Aviv Bergmana and Arturo Casadevall

    http://mbio.asm.org/content/1/5/e00212-10.
    full?sid=3927b57a-d112-452b-bbce-e1e1f4743e1d

15. Blood regulating body temperature http://www. medicalnewstoday.com/articles/196001.php

16. Digestive Disorders - National Institutes of Health, U.S. Department of Health and Human Services. Opportunities and Challenges in Digestive Diseases Research: Recommendations of the National Commission on Digestive Diseases. Bethesda, MD: National Institutes of Health; 2009. NIH Publication 08–6514

17. Islami, F., Boffetta, P., Ren, J.-S., Pedoeim, L., Khatib, D. and Kamangar, F. (2009), High-temperature beverages and foods and esophageal cancer risk—A systematic review. Int. J. Cancer, 125: 491–524. doi: 10.1002/ijc.24445

    http://onlinelibrary.wiley.com/doi/10.1002/ijc.24445/epdf

18. $100 Billion Annually on water http://pacinst.org/ issues/sustainable-water-management-local-to-global/ bottled-water/

19. American Water White Paper, Challenges in The Water Industry: The Tap Versus Bottled Water Debate http://www. water.com/files/TapVsBottle012609.pdf

20. Bisphenol A and Reproductive Health: Update of Experimental and Human Evidence, 2007–2013 Jackye Peretz,1 Lisa Vrooman,2 William A. Ricke,3 Patricia A. Hunt,2 Shelley Ehrlich,4 Russ Hauser,5 Vasantha Padmanabhan,6,7,8,9 Hugh S. Taylor,10 Shanna H. Swan,11 Catherine A. VandeVoort,12,13 and Jodi A. Flaws1

    http://ehp.niehs.nih.gov/wp-content/uploads/122/8/ ehp.1307728.pdf

21. Abstracts of Selected Bisphenol-A (BPA) Studies, Breast Cancer Fund, Prevention Starts Here http://www.breastcancerfund.org/assets/pdfs/tips-fact-sheets/bpa-abstracts.pdf

22. Columbia Water Center Earth Institute Columbia University, "Bottled Water." http://water.columbia.edu/?id=learn_more&navid=bottled_water

23. Bottled Water and Energy Fact Sheet http://pacinst.org/publication/bottled-water-and-energy-a-fact-sheet/

24. Consumer Guide to Water Filters How to find the right water filter for your home

    http://www.nrdc.org/water/drinking/gfilters.asp

25. Pur water filter http://www.purwater.com/why-filter

Chapter 7 – Essential Oils
Essential Oil definition - www.merriam-webster.com/dictionary/essential%20oil

1. Healing Power Beyond Medicine, pg., 288, Carol A. Wilson

2. Modern Essentials A Contemporary Guide to the Therapeutic Use of Essential Oils

3. Cleopatra Beauty Treatments http://health.howstuffworks.com/wellness/natural-medicine/aromatherapy/history-of-aromatherapy3.htm

4. History of EO's http://umm.edu/health/medical/altmed/treatment/aromatherapy

5. Hippocrates http://digitalhippocrates.org/

6. Healing Oil Charts

Essential Oil	Healing Properties	Spiritual Significance
Hyssop	Digestive Issues, Respiratory Infections, Urinary Tract Infections, Improve Circulation	http://www.webmd.com/ vitamins-supplements/ ingredientmono-258-hyssop.aspx? activeingredientid=258 &activeingredientname =hyssop http://www.webmd.com/ vitamins-supplements/ ingredientmono-258-hyssop.aspx? activeIngredientId=258 &activeIngredientName= hyssop&source=1
Myrrh	Skin Allergies, Gum Disease, Infection, Skin Wounds or Skin Problems	Book, http://www.webmd.com/ vitamins-supplements/ ingredientmono-570-myrrh.aspx? activeIngredientId=570& activeIngredientName=myrrh &source=1
Cinnamon	Antibacterial, Antifungal, Diabetes, Mold, Respiratory Infection, Warming	http://en.wikibooks.org/wiki/ Complete_Guide_to_Essential_ Oils/A_to_Z_of_essential_ oils/Cinnamon http://www.webmd.com/ vitamins-supplements/ ingredientmono-330-Cinnamon+CINNAMON +bark.aspx?activeIngredientId= 330&activeIngredientName= Cinnamon+(CINNAMON +bark)&source=2

Pine	Antibacterial, Disinfectant, Antiseptic, Natural Deodorizer, Influenza, Herpes Simplex Type 1 & 2, E. Coli, Candida Albicans, Lower Respiratory Tract Swelling, Inflammation, Cold, Cough, Bronchitis, Fevers, Blood Pressure, Stuffy Nose, Muscle Pain and Nerve Pain	Wikipedia http://biblehub.com/topical/p/pine.htm http://biblehub.com/topical/p/pine.htm http://www.webmd.com/vitamins-supplements/ingredientmono-101-pine.aspx?activeIngredientId=101&activeIngredientName=pine&source=1
Cedarwood	Antifungal, Disinfectant, Household Cleaning, Skin Care, Alopecia, Insect Repellent	http://www.webmd.com/vitamins-supplements/ingredientmono-1119-Cedarwood+oil+ATLANTIC+CEDAR.aspx?activeIngredientId=1119&activeIngredientName=Cedarwood+oil+(ATLANTIC+CEDAR)&source=2
Frankincense	Osteoarthritis, Rheumatoid Arthritis, Joint Pain, Bursitis, Tendonitis, Ulcerative Colitis, Abdominal Pain, Hay Fever, Sore Throat, Syphilis, Menstruation, Pimples and Cancer	http://www.webmd.com/vitamins-supplements/ingredientmono-63-frankincense.aspx?activeIngredientId=63&activeIngredientName=frankincense&source=1
Myrtle	Antifungal, Antibacterial, Treating Lung Infections, Bronchitis, Whooping Cough, Tuberculosis, Bladder Conditions, Diarrhea and Worms	http://www.webmd.com/vitamins-supplements/ingredientmono-556-myrtle.aspx?activeIngredientId=556&activeIngredientName=myrtle&source=1

Galbanum	Skin Wounds, Digestion Problems, Flatulence, Poor Appetite, Cough and Spasms	http://www.webmd.com/ vitamins-supplements/ ingredientmono-665-Galbanum. aspx?activeIngredientId= 665&activeIngredientName =Galbanum&source=1
Aloes (Sandalwood)	Common Cold, Cough, Bronchitis, Fever, Sore Mouth and Throat, Urinary Tract Infection, Liver Disease, Gallbladder Problems, Heatstroke, Headache, Conditions of the Heart and Blood Vessels (Cardiovascular Disease)	http://www.webmd.com/ vitamins-supplements/ ingredientmono-116-Sandalwood+WHITE+ SANDALWOOD. aspx?activeIngredientId= 116&activeIngredientName =Sandalwood+(WHITE+ SANDALWOOD)&source=2
Rose of Sharon	Stomach Irritation, Disorders of Circulation, Laxative, Diuretic, Upper Respiratory Tract Pain and Swelling, Heart and Nerve Diseases, Loss of Appetite, Colds, Fluid Retention	http://www.webmd.com/ vitamins-supplements/ ingredientmono-211-Hibiscus. aspx?activeIngredientId= 211&activeIngredientName= Hibiscus&source=1
Spikenard	Skin Disease Treatment, Coughs, Asthma, Arthritis, Loosen Congestion, Boost Tissue Regrowth and Promotes Sweating	http://www. biblestudytools.com/ dictionary/spikenard/ http://biblehub.com/topical/ s/spikenard.htm http://en.wikipedia.org/wiki/ Spikenard

7. Carrier Oil Definition http://en.wikipedia.org/wiki/Carrier_oil

8. Exploring Aromatherapy Safety Information https://www.naha.org/explore-aromatherapy/safety/ and https://www.naha.org/explore-aromatherapy/safety/

9. Limbic System http://en.wikipedia.org/wiki/Limbic_system

10. Quote prescription drugs http://www.skainfo.com/health_care_market_reports/2012_promotional_spending.pdf

    http://www.pewtrusts.org/en/research-and-analysis/fact-sheets/2013/11/11/persuading-the-prescribers-pharmaceutical-industry-marketing-and-its-influence-on-physicians-and-patients

11. $300 Billion annually http://www.who.int/trade/glossary/story073/en/

12. Injury Prevention & Control: Prescription Drug Overdose http://www.cdc.gov/drugoverdose/epidemic/index.html

13. Coma Recovery, Traumatic Brain Injury http://www.drugawareness.org/cnn-teen-in-coma-from-severe-brain-injury-recovers-with-alternatives/

14. ADHD http://www.brainbalancecenters.com/blog/2014/10/essential-oils-adhd/

15. National Health Statistics Report CDC http://www.cdc.gov/nchs/data/nhsr/nhsr079.pdf

16. Cleveland Clinic Among First In U.S. To Open Hospital-based Chinese Herbal Therapy Clinic, March 5, 2014 http://my.clevelandclinic.org/about-cleveland-clinic/newsroom/releases-videos-newsletters/2014-3-5-cleveland-clinic-among-first-in-the-us-to-open-hospital-based-chinese-herbal-therapy-clinic

Chapter 8 – Remember the Sabbath

Sabbath definition http://www.dictionary.reference.com/browse/Sabbath
1. Earth's Axis What if There Were No Seasons? Live Science http://www.livescience.com/18972-earth-seasons-tilt.html

2. American Institute of Stress http://americaninstituteofstress.org

3. American Psychological Association Why Sleep is Important What Happens When You Don't Get Enough http://www.apa.org/topics/sleep/why.aspx

4. National Heart, Lung Blood Institute Why Sleep is Important http://www.nhlbi.nih.gov/health/health-topics/topics/sdd/why

5. Sleep Disorders – National Sleep Foundation http://sleepfoundation.org/sleep-disorders-problems

6. How Much Sleep Do I Need? CDC http://www.cdc.gov/sleep/about_sleep/how_much_sleep.htm

Chapter 9 – Preserve & Protect Planet Earth
Preserve definition: https://www.google.com/webhp?sourceid=chrome-instant&rlz=1C1SNNT_enUS447&ion=1&espv=2&es_th=1&ie=UTF-8#es_th=1&q=preserve%20definition

1. Digital Receipts: Beyond The Green Benefit Digital receipts are going mainstream, fueled by stakeholder benefits that span from the consumer to the front office, Dec 2012 http://www.celerant.com/default/assets/File/Celerant_GreenReceipts_V1(1).pdf

2. BPA Printed Receipts - http://green.blogs.nytimes.com/2011/11/01/check-your-receipt-it-may-be-tainted/?_r=1

3. EPA Plastics - http://www.epa.gov/wastes/conserve/materials/plastics.htm

4. Reuseit Plastic Bag Pandemic www.reuseit.com/.../learn-more-facts-about-the-plastic-bag-pandemic.htm

5. Reducing Disposable Bag Pollution – Statistics http://www.citizenscampaign.org/campaigns/plastic-bags.asp

6. Ireland PlasTax http://www.nytimes.com/2008/02/02/world/europe/02bags.html?pagewanted=1&_r=3&sq=reusablebags&st=nyt&scp=1&

7. Other Countries banned plastic bags http://www.catholic.org/news/green/story.php?id=49191

8. Food Miles http://en.wikipedia.org/wiki/Food_miles#cite_note-8

9. Food, Fuel, and Freeways: An Iowa perspective on how far food travels, fuel usage, and greenhouse gas emissions http://ngfn.org/resources/ngfn-database/knowledge/food_mil.pdf Food Transport 1,500 miles - Pirog R, Pelt T Van, Enshayan K, Cook E. Food, Fuel, and Freeways: An Iowa Perspective on How Far Food Travels, Fuel Usage, and Greenhouse Gas Emissions. Ames, Iowa: Leopold Center for Sustainable Agriculture; 2001.

10. EPA 13% Green House Gas Emissions Food Recovery http://www.epa.gov/foodrecovery/

11. Climate change and health http://www.who.int/mediacentre/factsheets/fs266/en/

12. Food miles: How far your food travels has serious consequences for your health and the climate https://food-hub.org/files/resources/Food%20Miles.pdf

13. Know Your Farmer, Know Your Food 0 USDA http://www.usda.gov/documents/KYFCompass.pdf

14. Municipal Solid Waste - http://www.epa.gov/epawaste/nonhaz/municipal/

15. Landfills EPA http://www.epa.gov/osw/education/quest/ pdfs/unit2/chap4/u2-4_landfills.pdf

16. Natural Resource Defense Council - Paper Industry Laying Waste to North American Forests http://www.nrdc.org/land/ forests/tissue.asp

17. Statistics on paper towels - http://www.scgov.net/ sustainability

18. Statistics on paper towels http://1800recycling.com/

Chapter 10
Revolution definition - https://www.google.com/search?q= revolution+definition&rlz=1C1SNNT_ enUS447&oq=revolution+definition&aqs= chrome.0.0l6.3687j1j4&sourceid=chrome&es_sm=93&ie=UTF-8

Made in the USA
Middletown, DE
19 June 2021

42300022R00129